PRACTICING
PRIMARY HEALTH CARE
IN NURSING

PRACTICING PRIMARY HEALTH CARE IN NURSING

Caring for Populations

Edited by

Sandra B. Lewenson, EdD, RN, FAAN

Professor
Lienhard School of Nursing
Pace University
Pleasantville, NY

Marie Truglio-Londrigan, PhD, RN
Professor
Lienhard School of Nursing
Pace University
Pleasantville, NY

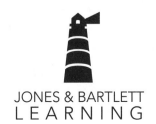

JONES & BARTLETT
L E A R N I N G

World Headquarters
Jones & Bartlett Learning
5 Wall Street
Burlington, MA 01803
978-443-5000
info@jblearning.com
www.jblearning.com

Jones & Bartlett Learning books and products are available through most bookstores and online booksellers. To contact Jones & Bartlett Learning directly, call 800-832-0034, fax 978-443-8000, or visit our website, www.jblearning.com.

Substantial discounts on bulk quantities of Jones & Bartlett Learning publications are available to corporations, professional associations, and other qualified organizations. For details and specific discount information, contact the special sales department at Jones & Bartlett Learning via the above contact information or send an email to specialsales@jblearning.com.

Production Credits
VP, Executive Publisher: David D. Cella
Executive Editor: Amanda Martin
Associate Acquisitions Editor: Rebecca Myrick
Editorial Assistant: Lauren Vaughn
Production Manager: Carolyn Rogers Pershouse
Senior Marketing Manager: Jennifer Scherzay
VP, Manufacturing and Inventory Control: Therese Connell
Composition: Cenveo® Publisher Services
Cover Design: Scott Moden
Rights & Media Specialist: Wes DeShano
Media Development Editor: Shannon Sheehan
Cover Images: top left: Courtesy of National Library of Medicine; top right: © Poznukhov Yuriy/Shutterstock; bottom left: Courtesy of Sandra Sheller 11th Street Family Health Services Center, College of Nursing and Health Professions, Drexel University; bottom right: Courtesy of National Library of Medicine.
Printing and Binding: Edwards Brothers Malloy
Cover Printing: Edwards Brothers Malloy

Library of Congress Cataloging-in-Publication Data
Names: Lewenson, Sandra, editor. | Truglio-Londrigan, Marie, editor.
Title: Practicing primary health care in nursing: caring for populations / [edited by] Sandra B. Lewenson, Marie Truglio-Londrigan.
Description: Burlington, MA: Jones & Bartlett Learning, [2017] | Includes bibliographical references and index.
Identifiers: LCCN 2015048786 | ISBN 9781284078107 (pbk.: alk. paper)
Subjects: | MESH: Nursing Care | Primary Health Care | Nurse's Role | Nursing
Classification: LCC RT51 | NLM WY 100.1 | DDC 610.73—dc23
LC record available at http://lccn.loc.gov/2015048786

6048

Printed in the United States of America
20 19 18 17 16   10 9 8 7 6 5 4 3 2 1

Contents

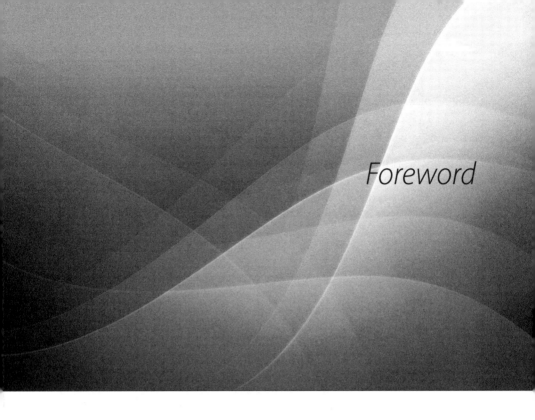

Foreword

Throughout my career as a nurse, educator, and researcher two main goals have been foundational to my work. These goals stem from my personal and professional experiences, and are framed from the perspective of my Latina background and my work in and with underserved communities. Specifically, my goals are (1) to increase public and community understanding of the scope and contributions of nursing in advancing health, and (2) to realize the potential of nursing in caring for the health of individuals and populations, especially those confronted with social, political, and economic challenges. In *Practicing Primary Health Care in Nursing: Caring for Populations*, Lewenson and Truglio-Londrigan comprehensively address these goals. They integrate their historical, public and community health, and shared decision-making expertise and lenses throughout the book to bring clarity to the issues of "who" and "how" to care for populations. In addition, they have amassed a number of contributors with a diversity of expertise and perspectives (e.g., historical, economic, public health, education, community, and social justice and advocacy) who address these goals by discerning the scope, issues, and approaches in caring for populations from a primary health care nursing perspective.

This book is timely as terms such as *population health, social determinants, health equity, primary care, primary health care, public health, community health, international health, global health,* and *culture of health*—to name a few—are being used interchangeably in contemporary social, health, and policy discourse. Although these concepts are related and differences may appear to be subtle nuances, how they are used to frame policy debates is of critical importance. Consistent with the perspective of the World Health Organization, primary health care is at the essence of health for all populations and is the organizing framework for this book. Chapter authors use this framework to illustrate the synergies among elements of primary care, primary health care, public health, global health, and promoting health equity locally and nationally, and demonstrate advocacy at the micro level (individuals and communities) and the macro level (national and global policy).

This book is timely as elements of the Affordable Care Act are being implemented. Policy debates and questions about "who" is best positioned to lead primary health care are made abundantly clear in this book—nurses! The chapters in this book examine the historical roots of primary health care and the role of nurses in both the United States and global context. We see the principles found within the Declaration of Alma-Ata in early public health nursing experiences, from Lillian Wald's Henry Street Settlement in New York City, to the American Red Cross Town and Country Nursing Service, to the work of public health nurses in the Indian Health Services on the Navajo reservation. Throughout the 20th century, nurses have shown leadership in primary health care in communities and at policy levels. Primary health care is not a shift for nursing; rather, it is part of a broader continuum of the professional role of nurses today. Contemporary nurses have led and designed models, including those designated as Edge Runners by the American Academy of Nursing—such as the Transitional Care Model and the Nurse Family Partnership—which are exemplars of nursing's continued commitment and success toward advancing primary health care. Historical and contemporary models incorporate core values of social justice, advocacy, interdisciplinary and multisectoral collaboration, and shared decision-making. In addition, these successful models and approaches incorporate strategies to address the multiple determinants of health including the environment, education, and housing within a community context. Further, many contemporary models have amassed extensive evidence to demonstrate that nurse-led approaches positively affect financial, patient, and family outcomes, indicating their value to both health care and population health. The numerous case studies and exemplars embedded in each chapter further demonstrate that nurses consistently have been, and are now, well positioned to lead efforts to advance primary health care through exemplary practice models, taking the lead in social and political advocacy.

While convincingly demonstrating the leadership of nurses in advancing primary health care, the authors also challenge nursing and its stated commitment to advocacy and social justice and the lack of ability, commitment, or action on these fronts. A number of useful frameworks and approaches, including economic and social value frameworks and community-based participatory action research, are presented in depth. Further, specific strategies to advance primary health care, such as community coalitions, partnerships, shared decision-making, advocacy, social justice, and cultural competency, provide a roadmap and skill set for addressing contemporary issues and challenges.

Each chapter contains a list of learning objectives, an exemplar or case study, and a set of reflective questions or learning activities. As such, this book is both foundational and an ideal reference for nursing and health-related history and policy-related courses. However, it also has great utility outside of the classroom. The historical perspective, links to contemporary context, and the multiple exemplars provide all nurses with the ability to articulate the scope and contributions of nursing in advancing health and to better prepare all nurses to advance primary health care for all.

Antonia M. Villarruel, PhD, RN, FAAN
Professor and Margaret Bond Simon Dean of Nursing
University of Pennsylvania School of Nursing

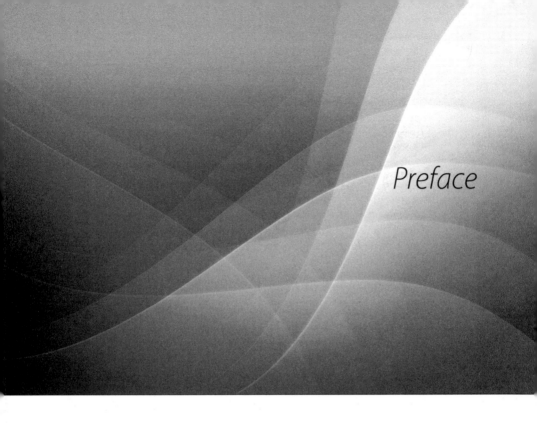

Preface

Practicing Primary Health Care in Nursing: Caring for Populations provides a unique examination of primary health care from a nursing perspective. The book presents the enduring relationship that nurses have had in pioneering primary health care with a population-based, interprofessional, and global perspective throughout the 20th and 21st centuries. Primary health care, as seen through the lens of nursing academics, historians, economists, and practitioners, places the profession's past practice and current visions into the ongoing health care debate in the United States. The multidimensional lens applied to the meaning of primary health care affords a way to educate nurses to understand and assume their rightful role in practicing within a primary health care framework, whether advocating health care policy in the political arena, developing coalitions with other professionals and community leaders, or engaging in shared decision-making activities in the community.

Practicing Primary Health Care in Nursing fills a void in the literature that all too often omits a nursing presence, a historical framework, and a philosophical perspective. In addition, it addresses the confusion surrounding the use of the term *primary health care*, which will help those engaged in education, practice, or research articulate and advocate better health care options and access for all. Building on nursing's central but often invisible role in primary health care, we provide a theoretical framework firmly rooted within the practice of nursing, both historically and contemporarily. Each chapter presents a view of primary health care from the contributing author's experience and uses a case study to explain the particular foci of that chapter.

Defining Primary Health Care

It is important to clarify the differences between the terms *primary health care, primary care, public health,* and *population-based care*—terms frequently used interchangeably in current healthcare debates. These terms serve as a guiding force for those seeking to implement the ideas of primary health care. Public health has a long tradition in the practice of social justice and population-based care. Population-based care, also a part of public health, is fundamental to the philosophy of primary health care. Primary care practitioners may use a population-based focus (Greenhalgh, 2007). The definition of primary health care continues to evolve within the context of health care in the United States as we struggle to separate these concepts.

The World Health Organization (WHO) first described primary health care in the Declaration of Alma-Ata in 1978. WHO's definition reflects a broader philosophical and holistic approach to health care that includes the contributing determinants of health that affect the health of populations. The Institute of Medicine (IOM, 2003) further describes primary health care as an intersectoral collaborative, which includes members from a variety of sectors in the community that have a stake in health care. These stakeholders may include members of the community, multiple disciplines, community organizations, public officials, academic settings, and corporations, with nurses participating equally. Representation from a population of interest may also serve as a participative member of this collaborative, informing the multiple players about the needs of their specific population. Primary health care uses shared decision-making and communication strategies that lead to improved population-based health outcomes. The health disparities identified in *Healthy People 2020* and addressed in the Patient Protection and Affordable Care Act (ACA), which seeks health equity for the entire U.S. population, resonates with the 1978 WHO definition of primary health care and the idea of "health for all." Nurses have had and continue to have a role in the development, practice, and evolution of providing primary health care services.

Primary Care Versus Primary Health Care

The term *primary health care* is often misunderstood and, as a result, misused. The term is used synonymously with "primary care," is blurred with "public health," and overlaps with "population-based care." Primary care does not reflect the totality of primary health care; rather, it is a point-of-care service model in which a health care provider, such as a nurse practitioner, midwife, or physician, meets with a patient in any setting in which care is rendered. Primary care owns "cultural authority and social legitimacy" (De Ville & Novick, 2011, p. 106), making this term more acceptable and used more often than primary health care in health care debates. As a result, it is difficult to shift our views to the broader and more abstract definition of primary health care (Truglio-Londrigan, Singleton, Lewenson, & Lopez, 2013). Public health nursing shares many of the underpinnings of primary health care and has been conceived as a "cousin" of primary health care (Greenhalgh, 2007, p. xi). A public health model, however, is not as abstract as primary health care seems to be and is more of a point-of-care model, albeit the point of care may be with a population.

Various models of care may fit within and aspire to provide primary health care. The concepts embedded in the philosophy of primary health care—shared decision-making, collaboration, social justice, community orientation, access for all citizens, and equity of services—may permeate primary care, public health, and population-based care, depending on how and if they are operationalized. A nurse practitioner may be caring for individuals and families but may not make the connection that those individuals and families are part of a larger population and as such miss valuable opportunities to develop initiatives to address population-based issues. For example, the nurse who makes home visits to a vulnerable older adult and sees depression in the client, if practicing with a primary health care perspective, would frame the intervention accordingly. This would include framing this one person's issue as a population-based issue. By looking at this as a population-based issue, the nurse may also work toward strengthening social supports and networks in the community. More importantly, without using the social determinants of health in the intervention, the practitioner may not address where the patient lives, works, and plays (Lavizzo-Mourey, 2015).

In the institution where we work now as academics, we offer master's- and doctoral-level courses in primary health care. Explaining the definition and practice of primary health care nursing can be challenging, but by the end of the semester we see the larger and more inclusive definition of primary health care become meaningful to our students and integrated into their practice. To help our students and the larger nursing audience who will read this book, we provide a variety of perspectives in each chapter highlighting various parts of the definition and meanings that reflect primary health care. The case studies, as well as the activities at the end of the chapters, provide real-life examples that foster creative and critical thinking toward achieving health for all. Each contributing author places her or his own perspective and experience on this broad concept, thus allowing for intellectual and practical flexibility.

The Editors' Perspectives

Both of us bring our unique understanding and perspective to the topic of primary health care. Sandra B. Lewenson brings a historical dimension to this discussion, examining how nurses have addressed health disparities in populations that led to changes in intervention strategies and better healthcare outcomes. She uses historical research to understand the ways nurses have participated in healthcare reform efforts over time. For example, she describes the early public health nursing leader Lillian Wald and her nursing colleagues' response to the human condition during the early part of the 20th century. Wald wrote in 1915 about her transformative experience while teaching a class on the Lower East Side of New York City that led to the development of nurse-managed intervention strategies in urban and rural settings in this county and abroad. Wald (1915) wrote:

> The child led me on through a tenement hallway where open and unscreened closets were promiscuously used by men and women, up into a rear tenement, by slimy steps whose accumulated dirt was augmented that day by the mud of the streets and finally into the sickroom... the odors which assailed me from every side. Through Hester and Division streets we went to the end of Ludlow; past odorous fishstands, for streets were a market place, unregulated, unsupervised, unclean; past evil-smelling, uncovered garbage cans; and perhaps worst of all, where so many little children played... although the family of 7 shared their two rooms with boarders... and although the sick woman lay on a wretched, unclean bed, soiled with a hemorrhage two days old, they were not degraded human beings. (p. 6)

Wald's commitment to the underserved in the Lower East Side tenements of New York City permeated the early 20th century efforts of public health nurses to improve health for all. Her work and that of her colleagues serves as a beacon for Lewenson. History frames Lewenson's conception of primary health care and offers depth and breadth to enduring and contemporary health care issues. Many of the authors selected to contribute to this work use their own historical research to exemplify a particular current issue in primary health care.

Marie Truglio-Londrigan's vision of primary health care has grown out of her long career in public health nursing. Her practice has been based on a belief that health care is truly a working partnership, whether that partnership is between her and an individual, a family, or a population. The significance of this partnership is in the work that builds up to shared decision-making as the collective engages in identification of the problem and in building interventions toward the resolution. Her research in a community setting study on shared decision-making with older adults highlights these ideas. Truglio-Londrigan saw the importance of joining with the older adults in identification of the population-based problems as seen by the population, exploration of the needed interventions as seen by the population, and the implementation of the interventions driven by the population, as well as the evaluation. Truglio-Londrigan saw the need for community-based participatory research with the key word being *action*. Action by the people serves to enhance their own personal capital and empowerment.

We both share similar stories in our practice as public health nurses. We have witnessed the effects of poverty in single-family households, food insecurity when families lack money for food or live in neighborhoods where food sources are scarce, and inadequate housing for families who live in communities with an absence of affordable living options. These are just three of the social determinants of health many of the most vulnerable among us face. A primary health care focus explores different kinds of solutions than those typically applied within a primary care or population-based care point-of-service delivery model. Nurses who practice with a primary health care focus recognize that to ensure healthy nutrition, for example, might mean more than educating the family about healthy nutrition. It may mean helping the family obtain the food by working with communities to encourage ways to bring food stores into the neighborhood that carry healthy options such as fresh fruits and vegetables and other sustainable food sources found in local gardens developed and nurtured by people in the community, and also supporting legislation that continues to provide healthy food for those under a certain income level. The context in which care is provided becomes part of the nursing assessment, plan, intervention, and evaluation.

Our understanding of primary health care also informs our practice as nurse educators. The ideas related to primary health care have always been a part of the philosophy and curriculum of the Lienhard School of Nursing. Both undergraduate and graduate courses in some ways infused the ideas of primary health care. When the graduate faculty developed a new master's core curriculum, there was a conscious effort to use the terms embedded in primary health care in each of the core courses, as well as to develop a signature course devoted solely to this concept.

Yet the paucity of scholarship on a nursing perspective in this area made the process of teaching these courses challenging. We saw a need for clear definitions and recognition that nursing plays an important role in the implementation of primary health care, especially as the Affordable Care Act expands opportunities for nurses. In fact, while finishing the second edition of *Public Health Nursing: Practicing Population-Based Care*, we realized we needed to include a chapter about primary health care. Truglio-Londrigan, Singleton, Lewenson, and Lopez (2013) saw this chapter as a conversation that enabled us to articulate the meaning of primary health care in relation to nursing practice in the United States. What began as a conversation later morphed into this book, which brings together our ideas about practice, teaching/learning, research, and primary health care.

Audience

Practicing Primary Health Care in Nursing offers nursing educational programs a way to broaden their curricula to encompass the concepts of primary health care and population-based care within their coursework. Chapters include a nursing focus within a perspective of primary health care. The integral role of nursing as a member of the intersectoral collaborative resonates throughout this text, emphasizing the essential role and value of nursing as recognized by the WHO, the IOM, and the current U.S. healthcare reform legislation. In addition, nurses and other healthcare providers may find this book useful as they use the language of primary health care to inform their practice. They will see their work framed in a broader perspective, which in turn provides the tools and terms needed in political advocacy.

Practicing Primary Health Care in Nursing

Chapter 1, "Historical Exemplars in Nursing," by Sandra B. Lewenson, explores the relatively unknown American Red Cross Town and Country Nursing Service, which provided public health nursing services to small cities and towns in rural America. Nurses built coalitions and collaborated with community leaders in rural settings to provide health care in the community. This chapter illustrates how the actions of one community between 1915–1917 reflects the practice of primary health care today.

In Chapter 2, "Awakening of an Idea," Kathleen M. Nokes describes how the philosophy of primary health care (PHC) emerged in South Africa prior to the 1940s. The country was plagued by apartheid policies, poor infrastructure, and little access to care, which produced poor health outcomes. Two physicians were influential in establishing comprehensive health service centers in South Africa that used a team-based approach. These centers were an early precursor to the World Health Organization's (WHO) Declaration of Alma-Ata in 1978 where the term *primary health care* was formalized.

In Chapter 3, "Nursing's Role in Building a Culture of Health," Susan B. Hassmiller discusses the disparities of health care in the United States and presents an idea for addressing these disparities in an alternative way. The Robert Wood Johnson Foundation promotes the campaign for a Culture of Health, which Hassmiller describes in this chapter. Hassmiller explores the leadership role of nurses in the evolving U.S. healthcare system as they individually and collectively engage in the process of leading change and advancing the health of all of the people.

Chapter 4, "Social Justice, Nursing Advocacy, and Health Inequities," by Selina A. Mohammed, Christine A. Stevens, Mabel Ezeonwu, and Cheryl L. Cooke, focuses on social justice and nursing advocacy. Throughout the chapter, the authors clarify the role of health professionals in primary health care and underscore the need for healthcare providers to work toward health equity through social justice, advocacy, collaboration, and ethical decision-making. Social, political, economic, and environmental factors are determinants of health that can be barriers to social justice. Advocacy facilitates social justice, and nursing practice is pivotal in ensuring these gains.

In Chapter 5, "The Economics of Caring for Populations," Donna M. Nickitas discusses the economic implications of caring for populations using a nursing social and economic value framework. Introducing the social determinants of health, she challenges us to focus on the vulnerable and access to care with three aims: (1) improving the experience of care, (2) improving the health of populations, and (3) reducing per capita costs of health care. Nickitas illustrates the need for nursing to understand and apply an economic perspective when examining primary health care.

In Chapter 6, "Coalitions, Partnerships, and Shared Decision-Making," Marie Truglio-Londrigan introduces various types of community coalitions and describes the outcomes of these initiatives, with specific emphasis on the Community Coalition Action Theory (CCAT). She illustrates the importance of coalitions from the perspective of the active engagement of the people in the communities, which leads to their empowerment. Truglio-Londrigan introduces multiple case studies to highlight the meaning of coalitions in health care.

In Chapter 7, "I Told Them, Leave It Alone; It's OUR Center," nurse historian Linda Maldonado brings history to life when recounting nurse-midwife Ruth Lubic's lifelong advocacy in developing community-based primary health care birthing centers in New York in the 1970s, and more recently advocating for the Family Health and Birth Center in Washington, D.C. The skills Lubic needed to create these centers included the ability to work collaboratively within the community, to be responsive to the various stakeholders, to keep data related to health care outcomes and cost effectiveness, and above all, the ability to create a safe and healthy environment for mothers and babies. This chapter reflects how advocacy intersects with a primary health care philosophy in action.

In Chapter 8, "Integrated Health Care Without Walls," Judith Lloyd Storfjell, Lucy N. Marion, and Emily Brigell describe using telehealth with the seriously mentally ill to support this population. Through a collaboration between the University of Illinois at Chicago College of Nursing (UIC CON) and Thresholds, the leading freestanding psychiatric rehabilitation agency in Illinois, integrated primary and mental health care has been provided to individuals with serious mental illness since 1998. What started as a half-day clinic at one Thresholds site evolved into three full-time, nurse-managed health clinics staffed primarily by UIC CON faculty advanced practice nurses. The health care team uses a primary health care approach with comprehensive, evidence-based, integrated primary and mental health care strategies that includes telehealth technology.

Any text about primary health care would be remiss without including a global perspective. In Chapter 9, "Global Nursing," Majeda M. El-Banna and Carol Lang provide a global perspective starting with the United Nations Millennium Development Goals, introduced in 2000, which were specifically developed to reduce poverty, hunger, and disease by the year 2015. They introduce us to the Institute for Health Metrics and Evaluation's Global

Burden of Disease (GBD) database, which compiles comparative data to identify trends in health worldwide. Compelling case studies reflect the needs of both developed and developing countries. The call for global health nurses requires curriculum infused with the ideas of primary health care, which "are key components in delivering health services to all."

In Chapter 10, "Culturally Sensitive Primary Health Care Interventions," Arlene W. Keeling, Brigid Lusk, and Pamela K. Kulbok explore the meaning of culture both historically and contemporarily. On a Navajo reservation from the 1920s until 1950 nurses learned how to work together with the Navajo population to build trust that led to acceptance of care. The second exemplar looks at the care provided for cancer patients post-mastectomy in the mid-20th century. Both historical exemplars took place almost 30 years prior to the Declaration of Alma-Ata, yet the nurses' care addressed gender inequalities as well as racial inequalities in American culture. The third exemplar illustrates a community participation model built on principles of community-based participatory research that is synergistic with primary health care. In addition, current technologies such as mapping and photovoic enabled public health nurses and their community partners to identify geographic trends over time and to target interventions. These three examples trace the importance of cultural competence in a PHC practice over time and space.

In Chapter 11, "Community-Based Participatory Research and Primary Health Care," Carol Roye and Marie Truglio-Londrigan describe a research project Roye completed in the 1980s. The findings of her project provided data for her practice, but it raised additional questions. If participants had assumed a more active role, she realized that her outcomes might have been different. This chapter defines the steps involved in community-based participatory research (CBPR) and explains how it supports nurses working within a philosophy of primary health care. Ethical challenges researchers using this method may encounter are also discussed. Although some may argue that health care providers know best as a result of their education, this chapter illustrates how both the consumer of health care and the provider, working in concert, can learn from each other throughout the research process.

Primary health care serves as a philosophical beacon for our practice, research, and education. Each of these chapters reflects the essential elements of primary health care as outlined in the Declaration of Alma-Ata. As you read these chapters, we ask you to reflect on your ideas, beliefs, and values about health care. We encourage you to become fluent in the broader conversation and comfortable with the actions needed to create a healthier nation.

Sandra B. Lewenson
Marie Truglio-Londrigan

References

De Ville, K. & Novick, L. (2011). Swimming upstream? Patient Protections and Affordable Care Act and the cultural ascendancy of public health. *Journal of Public Health Management and Practice, 17*(2), 102–109.

Greenhalgh, T. (2007). *Primary health care: Theory and practice.* Malden, MA: Blackwell Publishing.

Institute of Medicine. (2003). *The future of the public's health in the 21st century.* Washington, DC: National Academies Presss.

Lavizzo-Mourey, R. (2015). In it together—Building a culture of health. Retrieved from http://www.rwjf.org/en/about-rwjf/annual-reports/presidents-message-2015.html

Truglio-Londrigan, M., Singleton, J., Lewenson, S. B., & Lopez, L. (2013). Conversation about primary health care. In *Public health nursing: Practicing population-based care* (2nd ed., pp. 399–411). Burlington, MA: Jones & Bartlett Learning.

Wald, L. D. (1915). *The house on Henry Street.* New York, New York: Henry Holt and Company.

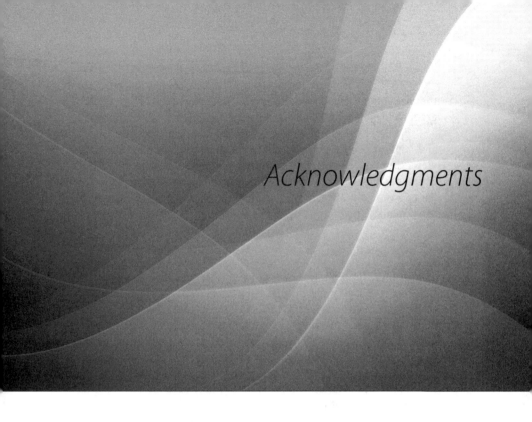

Acknowledgments

Sandra B. Lewenson

Acknowledging all that came before the planning and writing of this book is daunting. My colleague Marie Truglio-Londrigan, who was willing to meet on a weekly basis, deserves credit for her endurance, vision, and insight. Thank you to our publishers at Jones & Bartlett Learning who risked publishing a book devoted solely to primary health care. Our students who every semester learned to reconceive their worldview about health care have contributed greatly to the genesis and design of this book. To Donna Avanecean, our graduate assistant and herself a student in the Doctor of Nursing Practice program at our school, we appreciate your expertise and support. To our colleague Andréa Sonenberg, who participated in the early conceptualization of the book, and to our outstanding contributors, we owe a great debt for helping us to realize this text. Each and every author rose to the challenge of creating a chapter that examined this particular way of envisioning health care for all. They gave of their time, their ideas, and their faith in us generously to create a book that we hope will resonate with nurses, educators, and students in the years ahead. I also must acknowledge all the nurses of the past who saw the need to provide access to care for all, even before the term *primary health care* was coined. The ideas for this book come from so many sources, and as my colleague and coeditor Marie notes, the ideas about primary health care have emanated from the work of our graduate department faculty as well.

Finally, I could not have participated in this project without the love and support of my family. My husband, Richard, a dentist who shares my views about health care, has supported this project from its very beginning. My daughters, my sons-in-law, and our sweet granddaughters, Georgia, Sarah, Pearl, and Mira, have contributed to my understanding about health care. Thank you all.

Marie Truglio-Londrigan

The idea for this book is the result of decades of wondering about primary health care. My awareness of the essential elements of what became known as primary health care began prior to the Declaration of Alma-Ata as I embarked on my preparation for nursing at The City University of New York, Lehman College. Integration of these essential elements into this nursing program occurred because of the vision of the nursing faculty[1] at that time. I have been fortunate in my professional life to continually come in contact with men and woman who not only practice according to these central elements but live their lives that way.

The faculty at Pace University, the College of Health Professions, Lienhard School of Nursing saw and continues to see the ideas and values of primary health care as critical to the profession and to the health of the people of this nation, and because of this has placed primary health care at the core of their vision and mission. Thus, the stage was set for development of a text on primary health care. I thank Sandra B. Lewenson, my partner in writing this book. Her ideas and support throughout this project were invaluable, and she is an extraordinary mentor. I also wish to acknowledge my colleagues as the conversations we have shared over the years continually astound me. The ideas that are born in conversation truly exemplify the essential elements of primary health care and provide our students with the knowledge and skills to change our health care system—not only on the individual level but on family, community, and population levels as well—as we work to achieve health for all.

Finally, I wish to thank my husband, Michael Londrigan, and my children, Leah Pariso, Christopher Pariso, Paul Londrigan, and Jacqueline Jeselnik-Londrigan, for their constant support. They listen to me talk—on and on—about what I am writing even when they do not want to.

---

[1]Graduate faculty who developed the core courses using primary health care concepts included Catherine Concert, Martha Kelly, Lucille Ferrara, Marie Truglio-Londrigan, Sandra B. Lewenson, Joanne K. Singleton, Jason Slyer, Andréa Sonenberg, Renee McCloud-Sordjan, and Winifred C. Connerton.

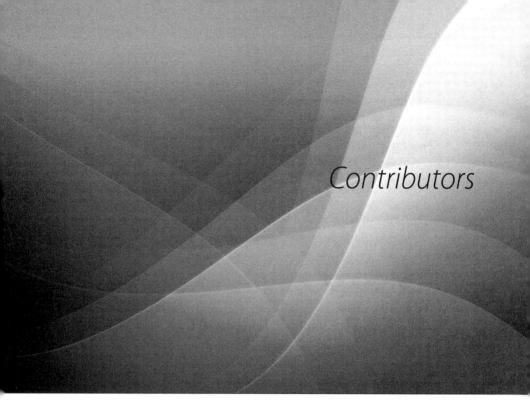

Contributors

Donna Avanecean, RN, FNP-BC, CNRN
APRN Comprehensive Epilepsy Center
Department of Neurology Hartford Hospital
Hartford, Connecticut

Yaa Boatemaa, MSN, FNP
Veterans Affairs
Brooklyn, New York

Emily Brigell, MS, RN
Director, Nurse Managed Clinics
Clinical Instructor
Department of Health Systems Science
University of Illinois at Chicago College of Nursing
Chicago, Illinois

Cheryl Cooke, PhD, RN
Associate Professor
Adjunct Associate Professor in Women and Gender Studies
University of Washington Bothell School of Nursing and Health Studies
Bothell, Washington

Majeda M. El-Banna, PhD, MSN, BSN, RN
Director of Nursing Advancement Program
Assistant Professor
The George Washington University School of Nursing
Ashburn, Virginia

Mabel Ezeonwu, PhD, RN
Assistant Professor
University of Washington Bothell School of Nursing and Health Sciences
Bothell, Washington

Susan B. Hassmiller, PhD, RN, FAAN
Robert Wood Johnson Foundation Senior Adviser for Nursing, and
Director, Future of Nursing Campaign for Action
Princeton, New Jersey

Arlene W. Keeling, PhD, RN, FAAN
Centennial Distinguished Professor of Nursing
Director of the Eleanor Crowder Bjoring Center for Historical Inquiry
University of Virginia School of Nursing
Charlottesville, Virginia

Pamela K. Kulbok, DNSc, RN, PHCNS-BC, FAAN
Theresa A. Thomas Professor of Nursing and Professor of Public Health Sciences
Coordinator of the Public Health Nursing Leadership Program
University of Virginia School of Nursing
Charlottesville, Virginia

Carol Lang, PhD, DHScN, MSN, BSN, RN
Associate Director Global Initiative Assistant Professor
The George Washington University School of Nursing
Ashburn, Virginia

Brigid Lusk, RN, PhD, FAAN
Adjunct Clinical Professor
Director, Midwest Nursing History Research Center
Department of Health Systems Science
University of Illinois at Chicago College of Nursing
Chicago, Illinois

Linda Maldonado PhD, RN
Assistant Professor
Villanova University College of Nursing
Villanova, Pennsylvania

Lucy N. Marion, PhD, RN, FAAN, FAANP
Dean, Professor, and Kellette Distinguished Chair of Nursing
Augusta University College of Nursing
Augusta, Georgia

Yvette Melendez, BA, MA
Vice President Government and Community Affairs
Hartford Healthcare, Hartford Hospital
Hartford, Connecticut

Selina A. Mohammed, PhD, MPH, RN
Associate Professor
University of Washington Bothell School of Nursing and Health Studies
Bothell, Washington

Donna M. Nickitas, PhD, RN, NEA-BC, CNE, FNAP, FAAN
Professor
Hunter College, City University of New York
Hunter-Bellevue School of Nursing
Executive Officer
Doctor of Philosophy in Nursing
Graduate Center, City University of New York
New York, New York
and
Editor
Nursing Economic$, The Journal for Health Care Leaders

Kathleen M. Nokes, PhD, RN, FAAN
Professor Emerita
Hunter College and Graduate Center, CUNY
New York, New York

Carol Roye, EdD, RN, CPNP, FAAN
Associate Dean for Faculty Scholarship
Professor Leinhard School of Nursing
Pace University
Pleasantville, New York

Christine Stevens, RN, PhD
Associate Professor
University of Washington, Tacoma
Nursing and Healthcare Leadership Program
Tacoma, Washington

Judith Lloyd Storfjell, PhD, RN, FAAN
Professor Emerita
University of Illinois at Chicago College of Nursing
Chicago, Illinois

Chapter 1

Historical Exemplars in Nursing

Sandra B. Lewenson

Chapter Objectives

By the end of this chapter, you will be able to:

1. Explore the historical dimensions of nursing and primary health care.
2. Analyze a historical public health nursing initiative in relation to the contemporary principles of primary health care.
3. Reflect on the enduring role public health nursing has played in providing access to health care.

Introduction

Long before the World Health Organization (WHO) defined primary health care in the 1978 *Declaration of Alma Ata*, nursing in the United States conformed to many of the principles found in that document. The ideals of health and social justice for all that permeate the definition of primary health care can be seen in the historical roots of public health nursing. Early 20th-century nursing pioneers long believed in the need to provide access to health care to all populations. These early pioneers, many part of the ever-expanding public health movement during that same period, sought collaborative relationships between and among nurses, physicians, dentists, philanthropists, and community activists. Although not all of health care history speaks to these holistic ideals rooted in early public health nursing experiences, many of these early "experiments"—for example, the American Red Cross Rural Nursing Service, later called the Town and Country (Buhler-Wilkerson, 1993)—demonstrated a concerted effort to provide populations in rural areas and small towns in America with access to quality health care services. Nurses, educated in the ideals of public health, led these early forays into what exemplifies the principles of primary health care today. They showcase what nurses and nursing leaders in the past saw as vital to the provision of care and can provide us today with important lessons.

Understanding nursing's past response to the health care needs of society requires study of the historical experiences of the profession, as well as acknowledgment of the evolutionary nature of health care. Noted contemporary nurse historians Fairman and D'Antonio (2013) explain that history helps us understand "continuity and change over time" (p. 346), especially when considering health care policy issues. Context and meanings change depending on interpretation and the orientation of the historian. Historian Joan Lynaugh's personal communication with Fairman and D'Antonio (2013) posits that all current issues have a past. This perspective helps us to see that matters like access to care, determinants of health, and social justice have a history that can offer meaning for us today and provide valuable evidence to guide contemporary practice. Knowledge of this history can help us as we struggle to understand nursing's role within the broader health care delivery system today, especially advocacy for and provision of primary health care services. For example, the current definition of the medical home calls for provision of continuous access to family-centered and culturally sensitive care (Keeling & Lewenson, 2013) and can be interpreted in a variety of ways by different professional groups. Physicians typically claim the leadership role in medical homes and are supported in these claims by insurance companies and politicians. Depending on the needs of the families served, however, other professional groups, such as nurses, may be better positioned to take on leadership and coordination of the care provided. During the early part of the 20th century, nurses had taken leadership roles in bringing both curative and preventive health care to families living in the community. These early historical nursing initiatives are valuable exemplars to aid our understanding of nursing in relation to primary health care (Keeling & Lewenson, 2013).

Historical Nursing Exemplar

This chapter examines a particular time in the early 20th century when community leaders in the rural upstate New York town of Red Hook sought to gain admittance into the newly formed American Red Cross Rural Nursing Service (renamed the Town and Country). In what was similar to today's concept of a medical home, the town of Red Hook applied to Town and Country to gain the nursing expertise this national organization offered to small towns and communities interested in providing access to care to their citizens. To understand Red Hook Nursing's 1916 application to Town and Country, a brief history of the origin of the American Red Cross's (ARC's) foray into the provision of access to rural health in America, as well as background on the community of Red Hook is provided. This illustrates how the actions of one community—Red Hook in Dutchess County— reflects the meaning used to describe primary health care today.

Background of Town and Country

Keeling and Lewenson (2013) refer to the start of the Henry Street Settlement in the Lower East Side of New York and the American Red Cross Town and Country when exploring the meaning of nursing's historical past in the provision of health care to underserved urban and rural populations. Both nurse-led initiatives were started by the public health nursing leader Lillian Wald, who transported public health nursing care (both curative and preventive) to populations that typically lacked access to care. In 1893, Wald began the Henry Street Settlement on the Lower East Side of New York City. She and her friend from nursing school, Mary Brewster, moved into the city's impoverished neighborhood that served as home to a diverse group of immigrants who settled in New York City in the late 19th and first half of the 20th century (Keeling & Lewenson, 2013). The settlement proved to be a place where "there has been a significant awakening on matters of social concerns, particularly those affecting the protection of children throughout society in general; and a new sense of responsibility has been aroused among men and women.... The Settlement is in itself an expression of this sense of responsibility" (Wald, 1915, p. v). The Henry Street Settlement success-fully provided nursing services to the population, first in the Lower East Side of New York, and later throughout New York City. The Henry Street Settle-ment also served as a clinical site for educational postgraduate programs to prepare nurses in public health experiences, such as the one started at Columbia University's Teachers College (Lewenson, 2015).

The success of the nurses at the Henry Street Settlement relied on collaborative community and political relationships. To make changes in health care policy, such as providing public health nurses in schools, Wald established relationships with community and political leaders and advocated the need for nurses to address the health care needs of schoolchildren (Lewenson & Nickitas, 2016). She successfully demonstrated the efficacy of public health nurses in city schools, which led to the integration of nursing services in municipal schools (Wald, 1915). Wald also lent her skills and expertise to the postgraduate program in public health that began in about 1912 at Teachers College at Columbia University. This program was designed to fulfill the additional educational requirement placed on any nurse who became a Red Cross Rural Public Health Nurse. It included both urban and rural public health experience and required collaboration with a variety of organizations, including Columbia, the Northern Westchester District Nursing Service, and other community settings (Lewenson, 2015; Wald, 1915).

Ideals of Social Justice Reflected

Wald's vision at Henry Street reflected many of the ideals of social justice promoted by the early 20th-century progressives, who were firmly rooted in the settlement house and other progressive era movements that sought equal rights and opportunities for all Americans (Drevdahl, Kneipp, Canales, & Dorcy, 2001). Jane Addams (1892), a leader in the settlement house movement and founder of the noted Hull House settlement in Chicago, explained, "The Settlement then, is an experimental effort to aid in the solution of the social and industrial problems which are engendered by the modern conditions of life in a great city." Wald's concept of a nurses' settlement, considered one of the first nursing settlement houses, reflected this philosophy. Her concepts of health care for all living in the community is something that we find in the late 20th- and early 21st-century ideals of primary health care.

Wald's vision to provide care to those living in urban centers expanded as she saw the need to provide this same care to rural populations throughout the country. Believing that nursing knowledge and skills legitimized nurses' work, Wald often spoke of the profession's role in social activism and social justice. Wald lived during a period of time when nursing's responsibility to social activism expanded in keeping with the national public health movement and other progressive era movements. In an address presented at the Red Cross convention in 1921, she described the changes she saw in nursing since 1893 when the term *public health nurse* was first applied to public health nurses and the collaborative role they played with others in the community. Wald (1921) explained,

> She has taken new vows and new obligations, and has expanded into something more important socially because her field, like her

education, has developed into the more comprehensive understanding of the relationship of herself and her profession to the physician, the hygienist, and the social worker. (p. 1)

In an address delivered earlier in 1913 at the newly formed National Organization of Public Health Nursing, Wald (1913) spoke of the

prophets among the nurses and among the students of social movements who see the veil lifted, and who know that the great army of nurses is educating the people, translating into simple terms the message of the expert and the scientist. The visiting nurses throughout the country have been reinspired to dignify and to lay true values upon their service, coveting for themselves the privilege of relieving pain, and linking with that century-cherished prerogative of women, the new note of education and civic duty. (p. 925)

Organizing the ARC Town and Country

Best known for her work establishing the Henry Street Settlement where public health nurses provided primary health care services to families living in the urban setting, Wald sought to bring similar care to those living in rural areas and in small towns throughout the United States. Such services included classes in health and hygiene, bedside care in the home, pre- and postnatal care, school nursing, classes in parenting, and other community-based activities. She envisioned using an existing national organization, the American Red Cross (ARC), to provide the necessary structure whereby public health nursing could be distributed throughout the country (Dock, Pickett, Clement, Fox, & Van Meter, 1922; Lewenson, 2015; Wald, 1921).

What began in November of 1912 as a 1-year experiment, with funding from the Rockefeller Foundation, a committee of socially minded philanthropists, physicians from the Public Health Service, and public health nursing leaders established standards for the practice and education of nurses in rural settings. Nursing leaders Lillian Wald, Annie Goodrich, Jane Delano, and Fannie Clement provided the ARC committee with their progressive ideas about recruitment, salaries, and education of rural public health nurses. With Fannie Clement appointed as superintendent of this new organization, she and the rest of the committee called for additional educational experiences in rural and urban public health—typically not taught in the 3-year hospital-based nurse training programs—for all Town and Country nurses. This educational requirement set in motion the establishment of 4- and 8-month postgraduate programs around the country that offered nurses courses in both rural and urban public health. Most famous of those schools was the program started at Teachers College, Columbia University, in New York City in 1912 (Lewenson, 2015). Rural public health nurses needed more education because of the nature of their work in isolated settings, which required that they have, among other things, good communication skills in order to develop collaborative relationships in the diverse communities in which they served.

By 1913, the successful outcomes of this first year of experimentation by the ARC Rural Nursing Service (as it was then called) included "ten affiliated associations, appointment of a nurse for supervisory work in the Metropolitan Life Insurance Company, the establishment of Teachers College course for rural nurses"(Minutes of the Fourth Meeting of the Committee on Rural Nursing, October 22, 1913). Renamed Town and Country after that first year, the service increased its scope to include small towns and rural communities. Nurses recruited to serve in these remote settings received additional education in all aspects of rural health, including courses in communication skills. These rural nurses needed expertise to negotiate with community leaders to facilitate health care services using whatever may already have existed within the community, such as a school board, a physician, or a visiting nurse service. Collaboration and coalition building were the hallmarks of rural public health nurses' ability to be successful in their work. These additional skills also set them apart from others in the profession and often created difficulty in the recruitment of nurses to rural settings.

Whether in urban or rural settings, public health nurses were part of a larger mission to help the immigrant population that came to America in the late 19th and early 20th century become "Americanized." In helping the immigrant learn how to become more "American," public health nurses helped immigrant populations live healthier lives and protected the rest of the citizens from illnesses that some believed would be spread by ignorance and poverty. Rose M. Ehrenfeld (1919), State Director of Tubercular Nursing, wrote about the evolution of public health nursing in the early part of the 20th century, and her words reflect the thinking of the day. Although not taking into account the issues related to diversity that nurses discuss in the 21st century, Ehrenfeld's ideas resonate with the ideals of primary health care:

> Public Health Nursing has become one of the strongest forces for Americanization, reaching into the homes and teaching foreign mothers how to interpret sanitary codes and to obey quarantine laws; how to select and use American foodstuffs with regard to nutritive value; how to raise the babies according to American customs and the demands of American climate. It represents the field of work that is reaching some of the "90 per cent of the sick outside institutions" with nursing care in their homes. It is extending to the masses pre-natal, tuberculosis, school, industrial, communicable disease and general community nursing; and, in so doing, represents the most important single factor in our national effort to check the slaughter of innocents by the kaiser of ignorance. It represents the instrument by which democracy's latest vision, namely, "equal opportunity for

health," is being practically applied and by which the light of modern science and the warmth of human sympathy are being spread into every corner of the world. (p. 18)

The Red Hook Nursing Association and the ARC Town and Country

In the historical example described here, we see how one rural community in upstate New York worked together as a community toward admission into the ARC Town and County between 1915 and 1917. Over 1 year's worth of correspondence between Mary Gerard Lewis, Corresponding Secretary of the Red Hook Nurses Association Nursing Committee, with Fannie Clement, the Superintendent of the Town and Country, illuminates one community's effort to develop a relationship with this national organization. Town and Country offered this community (and others like it) an opportunity to link an educated rural public health nurse with their community's effort to provide access to health care.

Description of the Red Hook Community

The town of Red Hook in the northwest part of Dutchess County in New York lies 85 miles north of the New York City metropolitan area (J Five Homes Realty, 2010). The area surrounding Red Hook included the villages of Annandale, Rhinebeck, Barrytown, and Poughkeepsie, all part of Dutchess County. The United States census shows the population in Red Hook in 1910 as 3,705 and in 1920 as 3,218. Rhinebeck had a population of 3,532 in 1910 and 2,770 in 1920. Poughkeepsie, one of the largest cities in the county, had a population of 27,936 in 1910, and 35,000 in 1920 (Zimm, Corning, Emsley, & Jewell, 1946, p. 355). The small towns seemed to show a decrease in population between 1910 and 1920, but the city of Poughkeepsie increased in size.

During the early 20th century, the population surrounding Red Hook included millionaire landowners, many of whom built large estates along the Hudson River that bordered the town. These estates, usually 300 to 400 acres or more, provided a source of employment for others living in the community. O'Neill Carr (2001) wrote that "many of the estate owners, following the tradition of their class in the 19th and early 20th centuries, sought to 'improve' the lives of their workers, and the surrounding community, primarily through religion and education" (p. 45). Names of wealthy families like Astor, Chanler, Aldrich, and Delano were connected to these estates and supported the tradition of social support to the community. The rest of the population of Red Hook and its environs included farmers and tenants of those farms who worked the land for their livelihood. Other groups worked in the county's industries, which included growing tobacco, cocoa, and violets as well as other seasonal industries like fishing and apple farming (Allen, 1925; State Charities Aid Association, 1915). The ethnic background of the community was mostly of German descent.

State Charities Aid Association 1915 Study

Most of the towns and villages in Dutchess County, except Rhinebeck, lacked the health care services many in the community believed were needed. Rhinebeck, the village next to Red Hook, established the Thompson House District Nursing Service in 1902 with only one nurse hired to care for their surgical, medical, obstetrical, and tuberculin cases (Waters, 1912). The Thompson House District received funding from Thomas Thompson, who had left more than $1 million in trust for the "relief of poor seamstresses and shop girls" in the towns of Brattleboro, Vermont, and Rhinebeck, New York (Waters, 1912, pp. 224–225). Out of this fund, hospitals and community nursing services were built in these two towns by 1912.

This early experience with a public health nurse in Rhinebeck showed the efficacy of using a public health nurse. Yet the people living in Dutchess County still lacked sufficient access to health care, both in the home and in hospitals (State Charities Aid Association, 1915; Weber, 1917). The health care organizations that existed worked in separate spheres; "their work was often unrelated and left important gaps to be filled" (Weber, 1917, p. 7). Concern for this lack of services led the State Charities Aid Association (1915) to conduct a study of the kinds of illnesses the population at large experienced and what kind of care was available to them. They selected four towns—Rhinebeck, Standford, Milan, and Clinton—as representative of the rural communities of Dutchess County (see **Figure 1-1**).

With the exception of Rhinebeck, the 1915 study found few if any of the towns in Dutchess County had access to a public health nurse or to rural physicians (State Charities Aid Association, 1915, p. 9). A door-to-door canvas of the families living in these four towns was made to see what kinds of sicknesses the families experienced, and how they addressed the care when sick. The study also showed the role that the rural public health nurse could play in care at home, in the hospital, or in the environment. For example, the study examines the environmental conditions that could lead to poor health, such as how many of the families they visited still maintained the "old-fashioned" privy vault and the use of private wells. The 1915 report noted, "It is to be observed in this connection that an epidemic in the village furnished 17 out of 29 cases of typhoid found by the investigator" (State Charities Aid Association, 1915, p. 9). The idea that environmental hazards related to draining the private privy into the water supply contributed to sickness and the health of the public is a concept still relevant today in primary health care.

The results of this study were used by the communities in Dutchess County to organize a Dutchess County Health Association in June 1916

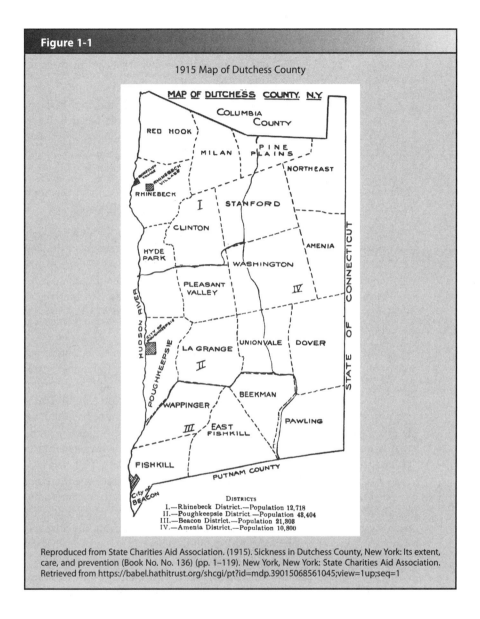

Figure 1-1

1915 Map of Dutchess County

MAP OF DUTCHESS COUNTY. N.Y.

COLUMBIA COUNTY

RED HOOK

MILAN

PINE PLAINS

NORTHEAST

RHINEBECK VILLAGE

RHINEBECK

I STANFORD

CLINTON

HYDE PARK

AMENIA

WASHINGTON

PLEASANT VALLEY

IV

HUDSON RIVER

CITY OF POUGHKEEPSIE

LA GRANGE

UNIONVALE DOVER

II

POUGHKEEPSIE

WAPPINGER

BEEKMAN

III EAST FISHKILL

PAWLING

FISHKILL

PUTNAM COUNTY

CITY OF BEACON

STATE OF CONNECTICUT

DISTRICTS
I.—Rhinebeck District.—Population 12,718
II.—Poughkeepsie District.—Population 43,404
III.—Beacon District.—Population 21,808
IV.—Amenia District.—Population 10,800

Reproduced from State Charities Aid Association. (1915). Sickness in Dutchess County, New York: Its extent, care, and prevention (Book No. No. 136) (pp. 1–119). New York, New York: State Charities Aid Association. Retrieved from https://babel.hathitrust.org/shcgi/pt?id=mdp.39015068561045;view=1up;seq=1

(Weber, 1917, p. 7), the same year that Red Hook explored establishment of their own Town and Country chapter of the ARC and the Red Hook Nursing Association. Town and Country supported the growth of individual town chapters, while also recognizing the value of one organizing chapter within the whole county. Clement (1916b) wrote to Lewis, noting that a Dutchess County chapter of the ARC already existed. In her letter, Clement wrote that even though the Dutchess County chapter existed and had a public health nurse, she still supported Red Hook and Annandale's effort to establish their own chapter and obtain their own rural public health nurse for their community. She suggested that the town chapter could be part of the larger chapter in the county but assured Lewis that the town would maintain control of the visiting nurse.

> Should it be possible to organize a Chapter in Annandale that might have direct charge of the visiting nurse work, it would be advisable to connect such a Chapter with the County organization so that in time of calls for relief the County Chapter with its various branches could act as the central organization. (Clement, 1916b)

Clement also responded to Lewis's letter regarding the county's plans for a tuberculosis nurse to work in the county. Clement (1916b) wrote,

> I shall be glad to learn more about the county plans for a tuberculosis nurse for as you say, it would be splendid to correlate the entire nursing activity of the County under the one organization. Various branches could be established in other sections through the county aside from Annandale and a visiting nurse might be supported in a number of districts on a plan similar to the one carried on by the Westchester District Nursing Association.

The Dutchess County Health Association seemed to be an outgrowth of the *Sickness in Dutchess County* report, published in September 1915. Although connections among the Dutchess County Health Association, Town and Country, and the Red Hook Nursing Association are not clearly delineated in these historical documents, some links seem to have existed. For example, Mrs. Richard Aldrich, one of the community organizers of the Red Hook Nursing Association, was also listed as the vice president of the citizens group that formed the Dutchess County Health Organization. Mrs. Richard Aldrich, whose name prior to her marriage was Margaret Livingston Chanler, was a lifelong resident of the town and a community leader with a history of volunteerism and support for the nascent nursing profession. In her younger years, she was a volunteer during the Spanish-American War, operating a field hospital in Puerto Rico, and later helped nursing pass a legislative bill in Washington, D.C., creating the Women's Army Nursing Corps at the turn of the century (personal communication, Wint Aldrich, January 27, 2015). In her community work in Red Hook, she referred to the State Charities Aid health survey as being an important impetus for the community to plan for a rural public health nurse. Her use of the data, as well as its use by others, illustrated an abiding interest in health care outcomes and access to that care for the population living in this rural section of New York (Chanler Aldrich, 1916).

Ideals of Primary Health Care Exemplified by Action

Red Hook's actions to establish much-needed nursing services in their community reflect today's ideals found in primary health care. Using current terms, community action, collaboration and coalition building, shared decision making, access to care, and community health education are just some of the activities the people of Red Hook undertook as they planned for and implemented public health nursing services in their community.

Community Action

On December 17, 1915, Fannie F. Clement, Superintendent of the Town and County sent a letter to Mary Gerard Lewis, corresponding secretary of the newly formed nursing committee from Annandale (a hamlet in the town of Red Hook), acknowledging Lewis's earlier inquiry sent to Jacob Schiff, philanthropist and on the board of the ARC, about the new rural public health nursing service called Town and Country (Clement, 1915). Schiff had forwarded Lewis's request for information to Clement, assuring Lewis that Clement would send both the application and a questionnaire for her to fill out in order to place the appropriate public health nurse in her town (see **Figure 1-2**). Clement also thanked Lewis, in her response, for offering her home to the Red Cross nurse to live as well as "in starting what would

Figure 1-2

Barrytown Minutes of Red Hook Nursing Association, May 2, 1916

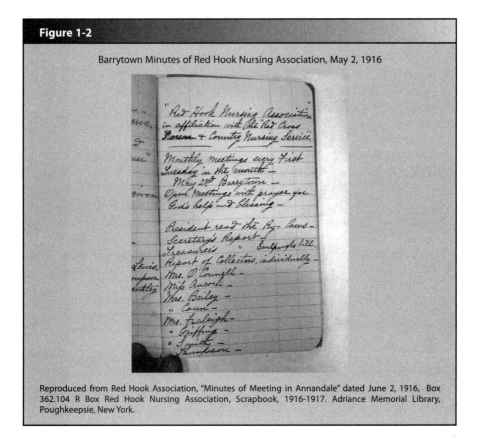

Reproduced from Red Hook Association, "Minutes of Meeting in Annandale" dated June 2, 1916, Box 362.104 R Box Red Hook Nursing Association, Scrapbook, 1916-1917. Adriance Memorial Library, Poughkeepsie, New York.

be a Community Center or a Neighborhood House for the surrounding country" (Clement, 1915).

Collaboration and Coalition Building

The citizens of Red Hook recognized that a concerted community effort was needed to bring public health nursing into their community (**Figure 1-3**). On February 11, 1916, the *Tivoli Times* published an article explaining the plan to start a nursing service and inviting the whole community to a planning meeting. The article stressed community support for this venture stating that "if this project is to succeed, the public must co-operate" (Red Cross rural nursing service, 1916). The nursing association would be responsible to care for those chronically ill in their community, as well as provide access to health care in a local dispensary. The minutes reflected these ideas, noting that "chronic cases to be visited by visiting nurse daily—whenever called" (Minutes of the Red Hook Nursing Association, April 4, 1916).

The nursing committee met monthly on every first Tuesday of the month to discuss the plans to establish a Red Hook Nursing Association

Figure 1-3

Unsigned Application for Affiliation with the American Red Cross Town and Country Nursing Service and Red Hook Nursing Association

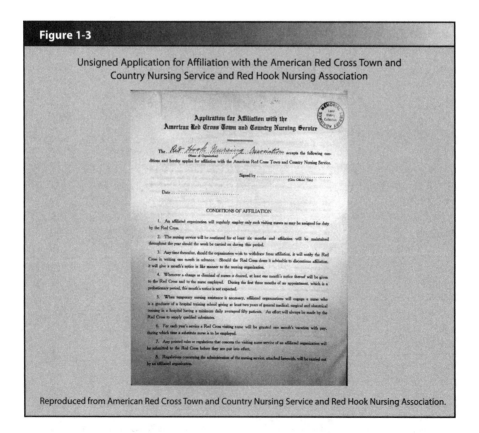

Reproduced from American Red Cross Town and Country Nursing Service and Red Hook Nursing Association.

and its affiliation with Town and County. Names listed in the meeting minutes included men and women from a variety of professions that committed time, energy, and money to support this venture. Community leaders Margaret Chanler Aldrich, Dr. C. A. Prichard (identified as the president of the committee), Mr. O. D. Lewis, Rev. J. Parks, and Mary Gerard Lewis (identified as the corresponding secretary) and other men and women in the community served in one capacity or another (Minutes of the Red Hook Nursing Association, May 2, 1916).

The minutes of these monthly meetings also reflected the larger community's input into the establishment of the Red Hook Nursing Association, especially in the organization of fundraising events. The minutes identified the various fundraising drives that would support the Red Hook Nursing Association and subsequent affiliation with Town and Country. For example, all families in the Red Hook Township would be given an "opportunity to subscribe" to the "R. H. N. A." (Minutes of the Red Hook Nursing Association, April 4, 1916). Families could buy subscriptions (usually one or two dollars) that gave them membership for the services of the Red Hook Nursing Association and supported hiring of the public health nurse. Those who had not yet subscribed would be sent cards with a follow-up from one of the members of the nursing committee. Various community members volunteered to collect the subscriptions from the families living in their village within the town of Red Hook. Other organizations held fundraising events, including "bag sales," "a strawberry festival," and a "camp fire girl's bake sale" (Minutes of the Red Hook Nursing Association, undated and unpaginated page in the brown minutes book). "Fetes" like the one given by Margaret Chanler Aldrich on May 27, 1916, on her estate, Rokeby, raised more than $300 (Red Hook Association, Minutes of Meeting in Annandale, June 2, 1916).

Shared Decision-Making

Shared decision-making could be found in the way that the Red Hook Nursing Association nursing committee called for the town to come together and participate in raising funds. Chanler Aldrich was especially vocal in her support of the development of Town and Country in Red Hook. In addition to her fundraising activities, Chanler Aldrich also wrote several letters to the editor in the *Tivoli Times* in support of her cause. She asked the community to participate in at least a Dollar Subscription drive so that the town could provide the much-needed services of the Red Cross rural visiting nurse. Without a rural visiting nurse, she felt that "Dutchess County will lag behind in business development, its girls and boys must accept modern life without modern safeguards, and our population will become few and weak. Our doctors cannot be our nurses" (Chanler Aldrich, 1916). Chanler Aldrich, along with other community leaders, saw the link between a healthy population and a better way of life for the population. And everyone, in all classes and walks of life, had a stake in health care.

Access to Care Through Affiliation

The nursing committee sought affiliation with the ARC and completed the necessary documents sent to them by Clement. The application included information about the town and their needs, and explained the requirements that they would need to meet. Nurses' salary, housing, and additional education requirements were all part of the application process and agreed to by the community. Community mass meetings about the affiliation were planned throughout 1916 and advertised in the local paper, the *Tivoli Times*. One such meeting was planned for Saturday afternoon, February 19, at 3:00 P.M. at the Masonic Hall. Miss Clement was to travel from Washington, D.C., to this town to explain more about the work of rural public health nurses. To ensure attendance, Mr. Harris Crockwell volunteered to take "a load of 20 persons for $4 to the meeting if they can be gotten together" (Red Cross rural nursing service, 1916). With use of the local media, including information about the monthly meetings and the plans for affiliation, the communities within the Red Hook Township banded together. The wealthier members along with those who could afford the price of the subscriptions were part of the effort to establish nursing services in their community.

Community Health Education

Fannie Clement wrote to Mary G. Lewis encouraging her to invite other rural Town and Country nurses to meet with the Red Hook community. These Town and Country nurses could inform the community about the kind of work that was done by rural public health nurses. In a letter sent by Clement to Lewis on January 4, 1916, she suggested that Lewis contact the Town and Country affiliate in Purchase, New York, located in nearby Westchester County. Miss Esther Harrison was the rural Red Cross nurse assigned to Purchase, and she could share her experiences at the meeting and show the "moving picture film" that had been developed by the ARC to illustrate the work of rural public health nurses (Clement, 1916a). On January 31, 1916, Caroline S. Read, president of the Purchase Nursing Association, wrote back to Lewis informing that Miss Harrison, their rural public health nurse, would be able to speak to the her group. Read wrote, however, that a time would need to be arranged in the future because at the present Miss Harrison's time was "very full with epidemics of measles and grippe" (Read, 1916). Miss Harrison, as Read wrote, held the trust of the community because she was "a very practical and vigorous worker as well as sympathetic." She also noted that Harrison was "not a good speaker, being shy and unable to speak very loud," but if the audience was not too large and they asked interesting questions, Miss Harrison would "forget herself and have wonderful accounts to give of the peoples' gratitude and willingness to follow as soon as they understand." By March 1916, Harrison's load must have lightened because she eventually met the community at a mass meeting and shared her stories. Harrison spoke of how she had to win the support of those in the Westchester community. She successfully gained their support when the community could see the care she provided to those who were ill and in her work with children in the schools (Address delivered at Red Cross meeting, 1916). Those who were unable to attend the mass meeting could read her speech, titled "Difficulty Attracting Rural Public Health Nurse," which was published in the *Tivoli Times*.

Attracting nurses with advanced postgraduate work to work in geographically isolated settings was challenging to Town and Country from its inception (Lewenson, 1915). To ensure the hiring of a permanent visiting nurse in Red Hook, Clement (1916a) wrote early on in the planning stage that at least 6-months' salary had to be guaranteed and at least 3 months' had to be deposited in the bank. In addition, a central location for the nurses' residence was important so that the nurse would be "within easy access to the greatest number of families." With the location in mind, the nursing committee also had to figure in the kind of transportation the visiting nurse would need that would give her the most access. Clement (1916c) wrote, "Your nurse, I am sure, will need a horse and buggy to visit her cases or else a horse, and then it will not make such a great deal of difference as to where she is located." With a plan to hire someone by June 1, 1916, the pressure to raise sufficient funds to support this venture was evident, prompting Clement to ask, "Have you tried to get each church to give a supper or some entertainment for the benefit of the nursing fund?" The Red Hook community eventually collected enough funds, and in the fall of 1916 (a few months past the June date) they hired the Town and Country nurse Margaret E. Ruba as their rural public health nurse (District nurse now engaged, n.d.). Clement (1916d) announced the establishment of Red Hook's new nursing service in the November 1916 edition of the *American Journal of Nursing* along with the expansion of other communities throughout the United States.

Health Care Outcomes

Outcomes of Ruba's early days in Red Hook were described in the December 8, 1916, edition of the *Tivoli Times*, noting that her examinations of children in school in four of the districts within Red Hook successfully identified problems with 184 children out of a total of 261 children. Some of the deficits she found in her assessment included dental and vision problems, enlarged tonsils, nasal obstruction, or other deformities. The aim of the Red Hook Nursing Association was to correct these problems. Within a short time, Ruba had made a total of 131 home visits and given 16 health-related talks to a variety of schools, organizations, and businesses (Large field for our Red Cross nurses' work, 1916). Her success led the town to consider hiring an additional rural nurse as well as to participate more fully in the Red Cross nursing service.

The war in Europe by this time had led several health care providers, nurses and physicians alike, to leave their communities and serve in the war effort. The necessity for a healthy population became even more apparent as the need for more public health nurses rose during this period. When the Red Hook Nursing Association began, local health care needs required ongoing vigilance by the community to continue on its trajectory of providing for a healthier population for all in the community.

Conclusion

The ARC Town and Country offered Americans a model of care that today we might call primary health care. The Red Hook community in Dutchess County successfully navigated the application process to this national organization, ultimately providing access to care to those living in the community. Affiliation with Town and Country illustrates how the early 20th-century ideals held by progressive community leaders and public health nursing activists informed and improved the health of their communities then, as they do for us today.

Chapter Activities

1. Explore the history of early public health initiatives in rural and urban communities and show how they relate to primary health care.
2. Discuss nursing leadership in primary health care in the United States from a historical perspective.

References

Addams, J. (1892, Summer). *The subjective necessity for social settlements.* Presented at the School of Applied Ethics in Plymouth, Massachusetts. Retrieved from So Just: Speeches on Social Justice, http://www.sojust.net/speeches/jane _addams_necessity.html

Address delivered at Red Cross meeting. (1916, March 3). *Tivoli Times.* Located in Adriance Memorial Library, Poughkeepsie, New York, Box 362.104 R Box Red Hook Nursing Association, Scrapbook, 1916–1917. Retrieved from Worldcat database, http://www.worldcat.org/identities/nc-red%20hook%20nursing%20 association%20red%20hook%20n%20y/

Allen, J. C. (1925, April). Field training for rural public health nurses: An experiment in Dutchess County, New York. *Teachers College Record,* 649–659.

Buhler-Wilkerson, K. (1993). Public health then and now: Bringing care to the people: Lillian Wald's legacy to public health nursing. *American Journal of Public Health, 83*(12), 1778–1782.

Chanler Aldrich, M. (1916, April 6). Red Cross rural nurse. [Letter to the Editor.] *Tivoli Times.* Located in Adriance Memorial Library, Poughkeepsie, New York, Box 362.104 R Box Red Hook Nursing Association, Scrapbook, 1916–1917. Retrieved from Worldcat database, http://www.worldcat.org /identities/nc-red%20hook%20nursing%20association%20red%20hook% 20n%20y/

Clement, F. F. (1915, December 17). *Letter from Fannie F. Clement to Miss Mary Gerard Lewis.* (Red Hook Nursing Association Records, Box 362.104 R.) Poughkeepsie, NY: Adriance Memorial Library.

Clement, F. F. (1916a, January 4). *Letter from Fannie F. Clement to Miss Mary Gerard Lewis.* (Red Hook Nursing Association Records, Box 362.104 R.) Poughkeepsie, NY: Adriance Memorial Library.

Clement, F. F. (1916b, January 11). *Letter from Fannie F. Clement to Miss Mary Gerard Lewis.* (Red Hook Nursing Association Records, Box 362.104 R.) Poughkeepsie, NY: Adriance Memorial Library.

Clement, F. F. (1916c, April 12). *Letter from Fannie F. Clement to Miss Mary Gerard Lewis.* (Red Hook Nursing Association Records, Box 362.104 R.) Poughkeepsie, NY: Adriance Memorial Library.

Clement, F. F. (1916d). Red Cross: Town and Country nursing service. *American Journal of Nursing, 17*(2), 147–149.

District nurse now engaged (n.d.). Located in Adriance Memorial Library, Poughkeepsie, New York, Box 362.104 R Box Red Hook Nursing Association, Scrapbook, 1916–1917. n.p. Retrieved from Worldcat database, http://www.worldcat .org/identities/nc-red%20hook%20nursing%20association%20red%20 hook%20n%20y/

Dock, L., Pickett, S. E., Clement, F. F., Fox, E., & Van Meter, A. R. (1922). *History of American Red Cross nursing.* New York: MacMillan Company.

Drevdahl, D., Kneipp, S. M., Canales, M. K., & Dorcy, K. S. 2001. Reinvesting in social justice: A capital idea for public health nursing? *Advances in Nursing Science, 24,* 19–31.

Ehrenfeld, R. M. (1919). The evolution of public health nursing. *American Journal of Nursing, 20*(1), 14–18. Retrieved from http://www.jstor.org/stable/3405424

Fairman, J., & D'Antonio, P. (2013). History counts: How history can help our understanding of health policy. *Nursing Outlook, 61,* 346–352.

J Five Homes Realty. (2010). Dutchess County, New York, Area Info. Retrieved from http://www.jfivehomes.com/area-information/dutchess-county/

Keeling, A., & Lewenson, S. B. (2013). A nursing historical perspective on the medical home: Impact on health care policy. *Nursing Outlook, 61*(5), 360–366. doi: http://dx.doi.org/10.1016/joutlook.2013.07.003

A large field for our Red Cross nurses' work. (1916, December 8). *Tivoli Times.* Located in Adriance Memorial Library, Poughkeepsie, New York, Box 362.104 R Box Red Hook Nursing Association, Scrapbook, 1916–1917. Retrieved from Worldcat database, http://www.worldcat.org/identities/nc-red%20 hook%20nursing%20association%20red%20hook%20n%20y/

Lewenson, S. (2015). Town and Country nursing: Community participation and nurse recruitment. In J. C. Kirchgessner & A. W. Keeling (Eds.), *Nursing rural America: Perspectives from the early 20th century* (pp. 1–19). New York, NY: Springer Publishing Company.

Lewenson, S. B., & Nickitas, D. J. (2016). Nursing's history of advocacy and action. In D. M. Nickitas, D. J. Middaugh, & N. Aries (Eds.), *Policy and politics for nurses and other health professionals: Advocacy and action* (2nd ed.). New York, NY: Springer Publishing.

Minutes of the Fourth Meeting of the Committee on Red Cross Rural Nursing, dated October 22, 1913, Rockefeller Sanitary Commission Microfilm, Reel 1, Folder 8, American Red Cross Town & Country Nursing Service 1912–1914, Rockefeller Archives, Pocantico, New York.

Minutes of the Red Hook Nursing Association, dated April 4, 1916, Box 362.104 R Box Red Hook Nursing Association, Scrapbook, 1916–1917. Poughkeepsie, NY: Adriance Memorial Library. Retrieved from Worldcat database, http:// www.worldcat.org/identities/nc-red%20hook%20nursing%20association%20 red%20hook%20n%20y/

Minutes of the Red Hook Nursing Association, dated May 2, 1916, Box 362.104 R Box Red Hook Nursing Association, Scrapbook, 1916–1917. Poughkeepsie, NY: Adriance Memorial Library. Retrieved from Worldcat database, http:// www.worldcat.org/identities/nc-red%20hook%20nursing%20association%20 red%20hook%20n%20y/

O'Neill Carr, C. (2001). *A brief history of Red Hook: The living past of a Hudson Valley community.* New York, NY: Wise Family Trust.

Read, C. S. (1916, January 31). *Letter from Caroline R. Read to Miss Mary Gerard Lewis.* (Red Hook Nursing Association Records, Box 362.104 R.) Poughkeepsie, NY: Adriance Memorial Library.

The Red Cross rural nursing service. (1916, February 11) *Tivoli Times.* Located in Adriance Memorial Library, Poughkeepsie, New York, Box 362.104 R Box Red Hook Nursing Association, Scrapbook, 1916–1917. Retrieved from Worldcat database, http://www.worldcat.org/identities/nc-red%20hook%20nursing% 20association%20red%20hook%20n%20y/

Red Hook Association, "Minutes of Meeting in Annandale" dated June 2, 1916, (Box 362.104 R Box Red Hook Nursing Association, Scrapbook, 1916–1917.) Poughkeepsie, NY: Adriance Memorial Library. Retrieved from Worldcat database, http://www.worldcat.org/identities/nc-red%20hook%20nursing% 20association%20red%20hook%20n%20y/

State Charities Aid Association. (1915). *Sickness in Dutchess County, New York: Its extent, care, and prevention* (Book No. 136; pp. 1–119). New York, NY: State Charities Aid Association. Retrieved from https://babel.hathitrust.org /shcgi/pt?id=mdp.39015068561045;view=1up;seq=1

Wald, L. D. (1913). Address by the president of the National Organization for Public Health Nursing. *American Journal of Nursing, 13*(12), 924–926.

Wald, L. D. (1915). *The house on Henry Street.* New York, NY: Henry Holt and Company.

Wald, L. D. (1921). Address at the Red Cross convention, Columbus, Ohio, October 6, 1921. *The Henry Street Nurse, 2*(10–11), 1–5. (New York Public Library, Lillian Wald Papers, Reel 25.)

Waters, Y. (1912). *Visiting nurses in the United States* (2nd ed.; pp. 224–225). New York, NY: Charities Publications Committee.

Weber, J. J. (1917). *A county at work at its health problems: A statement of accomplishment by the Dutchess County Health Association during the sixteen months August 1916 to December 1917 inc.* New York, NY: State Charities Aid Association. Retrieved from https://babel.hathitrust.org/shcgi/pt?id=mdp.39 015014861580;view=1up;seq=1

Zimm, L. H., Corning, R. A. E., Emsley, J. W., & Jewell, W. C. (1946). *Southeastern New York: A History of counties of Ulster, Dutchess, Orange, Rockland, and Putnam* (Vol. I). New York, NY: Lewis Historical Publishing Company.

Chapter 2

Awakening of an Idea: Principles of Primary Health Care in the Declaration of Alma-Ata

Kathleen M. Nokes

Chapter Objectives

By the end of this chapter, you will be able to:

1. Identify how the principles of primary health care evolved from a South African governmental attempt to meet the needs of underserved populations.
2. Identify the World Health Organization's principles of primary health care found in the Alma-Ata Declaration.
3. Explore the primary health care nursing practice within the World Health Organization.

Introduction

Organizations such as the Ministry of Health of South Africa and the Centers for Disease Control and Prevention (CDC) in the United States are charged with promoting the health of the populations in the countries where they are located. The health status of populations is seen as greatly influenced by determinants of health including: policy making; social and physical factors; access to health care; individual health behaviors; as well as biology and genetic factors (U.S. Department of Health and Human Services [USDHHS], 2015). Recognition of the importance of all of the determinants of health on the health of populations can be traced back to the prior origins of primary health care (PHC), formally articulated in the Alma-Ata Declaration in 1978. This chapter presents the historical origins of PHC in South Africa during the 1940s whose indigenous populations had significant burdens of disease and exemplifies one of the early forays into application of PHC principles. Finally, the chapter highlights nursing's global operationalization of PHC in practice.

Background

In 1940s the South African Ministry of Health piloted the Pholela Community Health Center (Pholela) to address the health needs of the population greatly affected by poverty and deprivation, especially those living in rural areas (Tollman, 1994). A report issued by Henry Gluckman, the chairperson of a 1942 National Health Services Commission, recommended that a National Health Service (NHS) be developed. The NHS would establish community centers throughout the country to meet the needs of the entire population regardless of financial means. The vision was to economically sustain an NHS that would ensure adequate medical, dental, nursing, and hospital services for *all* sections of the people of the Union of South Africa (Phillips, 2014).

Sidney and Emily Kark, South African medical doctors, were appointed to develop and expand the Pholela model in a variety of communities (Kark & Cassel, 2002). Pholela sought to provide treatment, prevention, and promotion in a team approach that included physicians, nurses, medical aid graduates, and trained community health assistants. The health assistants were specially trained to deliver educational programs to the community (Kark & Cassel, 1952; Tollman, 1994). The main function of the health assistants was to provide education to people living in communities during home visits. The ultimate goal of the education was to facilitate behavior change in people, families, and the population as a whole that would assist them to lead a better way of life and achieve good health (Kark & Cassel, 1952). Common issues experienced by the population at that time included poor infant mortality rates, chronic malnutrition, syphilis, tuberculosis, typhoid fever, smallpox, measles, and whooping cough.

Kark (as cited in Tollman, 1994) explained the centers would provide the following essential functions:

> curative and preventive services, including the following essential functions: (i) prevention and treatment of disease; (ii) health education, with particular reference to the organisation of maternal and child welfare services; (iii) local cooperation and community responsibility... the activities of the health centre were to be co-ordinated with those other local agencies such as the authorities responsible for agriculture and education. (p. 653)

Initially there was suspicion among leaders in the community. Chiefs, Headman, and the local people objected to not being part of the decision-making process and to the lack of inclusion of local people selected to be health assistants. The health center addressed these concerns by organizing meetings between teachers, community leaders, church members, and elders with the health center members. This community advocacy led to the appointment of local community people as community health workers (Tollman, 1994). This approach of working with the populations, in their communities, was a major method employed within these health centers to establish trust. In addition, health centers identified a need to engage in activities that would provide the health center with data about these specific communities. An example of this data was the household health census and family health records. Tollman (1994) noted that this type of information was recorded on indexed cards.

Due to the increasingly restrictive policies of the apartheid government, the Karks left the Pholela project after 6 years. This was stressed by Phillips (2014), who stated, "from the start health centers of this ilk were not popular among the mainstream medical profession; after the accession of apartheid-minded National Party to government in 1948, the idea enjoyed dwindling support in the topmost echelons of official power" (p. 1874). After election of a democratic government in South Africa in 1994, the Pholela Health Centers were revitalized, but challenges due to the enormous burdens of tuberculosis and HIV/AIDS made full implementation difficult (Phillips, 2014). In addition, key to the development of this South African initiative is a realization that considers the complexity of population health, which requires the mindful dedication of many professionals who practice in a multitude of sectors (Phillips, 2014; Yach & Tollman, 1993). Of paramount importance are the challenges that may manifest themselves as shifts in government policy either enhance PHC initiatives or create barriers (Yach & Tollman, 1993).

Due to the integral role of community involvement in the Pholela project, the Karks called it community-oriented primary health care, which is now known as PHC (Tollman, 1994). Understanding the origins of PHC in this one South African nation is significant for it tells the story of the development of the essential principles as they took shape and form years prior to the Alma-Ata Declaration. Some examples of these include: (a) identification of the essential functions established for the Pholela Health Center are in evidence within the definition of PHC and in the declaration itself; (b) recognition of the multiple determinants of health that place populations at risk; (c) importance of education for changing behavior; (d) delivery of care in the community where the people live; (e) partnering with the people so that they are active and engaged in conversation and decisions; (f) collaboration and cooperation between and among all sectors such as governments, organizations, professionals, and community members; and (g) data gathering for populations and communities that serves as evidence for the development of initiatives. According to an influential leader in population health, the Karks assembled the girders upon which the Alma-Ata Declaration rests (Susser, 1993) through the Pholela Health Centers. What the authors of this text note is the omission of nursing from this history. Historical research is currently being conducted that will shed light on the centrality of nursing's work, which has been invisible from broader historical perspectives.

World Health Organization

The United Nations was created in 1945 at the end of World War II (United Nations, n.d.). The World Health Organization (WHO) is the directing and coordinating authority for health within the United Nations. It is responsible for providing leadership on global health matters, shaping the health research agenda, setting norms and standards, articulating evidence-based policy options, providing technical support to countries, and monitoring and assessing health trends (WHO, n.d.).

Alma-Ata Declaration

In the 1960s and 1970s, the failure of single-disease programs, such as that of malaria, and the lack of coordination between disease-specific programs prompted countries to ask the WHO for help in building their health services. Many developing countries had recently made the transition from colonialism to independence and were facing the challenge of how to extend health services, which had been designed for colonial elites, to the general population. The Health Assembly of WHO and the Executive Board of the United Nations Children's Fund (UNICEF) held the International Conference on Primary Health Care in 1978 in Alma-Ata, capital of the Kazakh Soviet Socialist Republic (WHO, 1978). This conference was attended by delegations from 134 governments, including Senator Edward Kennedy and other representatives from the United States, as well as representatives of 67 United Nations organizations, specialized agencies, and nongovernmental organizations in official relations with WHO and UNICEF. During this conference PHC was defined as:

> essential health care made universally accessible to individuals and families in the community by means acceptable to them, through their full participation and at a cost that the community and country can

afford. It forms an integral part both of the country's health system of which it is the nucleus and of the overall social and economic development of the community. (WHO, 1978)*

The Declaration of Alma-Ata may be fully viewed in **Figure 2-1.**

Figure 2-1

Declaration of Alma-Ata

International Conference on Primary Health Care, Alma-Ata, USSR, 6-12 September 1978

The International Conference on Primary Health Care, meeting in Alma-Ata this twelfth day of September in the year Nineteen hundred and seventy-eight, expressing the need for urgent action by all governments, all health and development workers, and the world community to protect and promote the health of all the people of the world, hereby makes the following

Declaration:

I

The Conference strongly reaffirms that health, which is a state of complete physical, mental and social wellbeing, and not merely the absence of disease or infirmity, is a fundamental human right and that the attainment of the highest possible level of health is a most important world-wide social goal whose realization requires the action of many other social and economic sectors in addition to the health sector.

II

The existing gross inequality in the health status of the people particularly between developed and developing countries as well as within countries is politically, socially and economically unacceptable and is, therefore, of common concern to all countries.

III

Economic and social development, based on a New International Economic Order, is of basic importance to the fullest attainment of health for all and to the reduction of the gap between the health status of the developing and developed countries. The promotion and protection of the health of the people is essential to sustained economic and social development and contributes to a better quality of life and to world peace.

IV

The people have the right and duty to participate individually and collectively in the planning and implementation of their health care.

V

Governments have a responsibility for the health of their people which can be fulfilled only by the provision of adequate health and social measures. A main social target of governments, international organizations and the whole world community in the coming decades should be the attainment by all peoples of the world by the year 2000 of a level of health that will permit them to lead a socially and economically productive life. Primary health care is the key to attaining this target as part of development in the spirit of social justice.

(continues)

---

*Reprinted from World Health Organization. (1978). Declaration of Alma-Ata. Retrieved from http://www.who.int/publications/almaata_declaration_en.pdf?ua=1

VI

Primary health care is essential health care based on practical, scientifically sound and socially acceptable methods and technology made universally accessible to individuals and families in the community through their full participation and at a cost that the community and country can afford to maintain at every stage of their development in the spirit of self-reliance and self-determination. It forms an integral part both of the country's health system, of which it is the central function and main focus, and of the overall social and economic development of the community. It is the first level of contact of individuals, the family and community with the national health system bringing health care as close as possible to where people live and work, and constitutes the first element of a continuing health care process.

VII

Primary health care:

1. reflects and evolves from the economic conditions and sociocultural and political characteristics of the country and its communities and is based on the application of the relevant results of social, biomedical and health services research and public health experience;

2. addresses the main health problems in the community, providing promotive, preventive, curative and rehabilitative services accordingly;

3. includes at least: education concerning prevailing health problems and the methods of preventing and controlling them; promotion of food supply and proper nutrition; an adequate supply of safe water and basic sanitation; maternal and child health care, including family planning; immunization against the major infectious diseases; prevention and control of locally endemic diseases; appropriate treatment of common diseases and injuries; and provision of essential drugs;

4. involves, in addition to the health sector, all related sectors and aspects of national and community development, in particular agriculture, animal husbandry, food, industry, education, housing, public works, communications and other sectors; and demands the coordinated efforts of all those sectors;

5. requires and promotes maximum community and individual self-reliance and participation in the planning, organization, operation and control of primary health care, making fullest use of local, national and other available resources; and to this end develops through appropriate education the ability of communities to participate;

6. should be sustained by integrated, functional and mutually supportive referral systems, leading to the progressive improvement of comprehensive health care for all, and giving priority to those most in need;

7. relies, at local and referral levels, on health workers, including physicians, nurses, midwives, auxiliaries and community workers as applicable, as well as traditional practitioners as needed, suitably trained socially and technically to work as a health team and to respond to the expressed health needs of the community.

VIII

All governments should formulate national policies, strategies and plans of action to launch and sustain primary health care as part of a comprehensive national health system and in coordination with other sectors. To this end, it will be necessary to exercise political will, to mobilize the country's resources and to use available external resources rationally.

IX

All countries should cooperate in a spirit of partnership and service to ensure primary health care for all people since the attainment of health by people in any one country directly concerns and benefits every other country. In this context the joint WHO/UNICEF report on primary health care constitutes a solid basis for the further development and operation of primary health care throughout the world.

X

An acceptable level of health for all the people of the world by the year 2000 can be attained through a fuller and better use of the world's resources, a considerable part of which is now spent on armaments and military conflicts. A genuine policy of independence, peace, détente and disarmament could and should release additional resources that could well be devoted to peaceful aims and in particular to the acceleration of social and economic development of which primary health care, as an essential part, should be allotted its proper share. The International Conference on Primary Health Care calls for urgent and effective national and international action to develop and implement primary health care throughout the world and particularly in developing countries in a spirit of technical cooperation and in keeping with a New International Economic Order. It urges governments, WHO and UNICEF, and other international organizations, as well as multilateral and bilateral agencies, nongovernmental organizations, funding agencies, all health workers and the whole world community to support national and international commitment to primary health care and to channel increased technical and financial support to it, particularly in developing countries. The Conference calls on all the aforementioned to collaborate in introducing, developing and maintaining primary health care in accordance with the spirit and content of this Declaration.

Source: Reprinted from World Health Organization. (1978). Declaration of Alma-Ata. Retrieved from http://www.who.int/publications/almaata_declaration_en.pdf?ua=1

Current WHO Leadership Priorities

The WHO maintains its commitment to the Alma-Ata Declaration, and multiple initiatives can be explored on their website. For the purpose of this chapter, just a couple will be considered. For example, in 2008 the WHO published the document *Primary Health Care: Now More Than Ever*. This report clearly articulated the gaps in health and the inequities noted between countries and within countries. The report also articulated not only challenges we need to face but the reforms that need to be made. The report highlights the following needed reforms:

1. Universal Coverage Reforms
2. Service Delivery Reforms
3. Public Policy Reforms
4. Leadership Reforms

Table 2-1 provides greater detail on each of these reforms.

More recently, the WHO (2014) published the *Twelfth General Programme of Work*, and the vision for its work including priorities and directions that will take place between 2014 and 2019. Chapter 3 within this document focuses on leadership priorities that include: (1) advancing universal health coverage; (2) implementing the provisions of the International Health Regulations (2005), which relate to public health emergencies emerging from

Table 2-1	
WHO Primary Health Care Now More Than Ever: Reforms	
Universal Coverage Reform	Health systems must contribute to health equity, social justice, and focus on universal access.
Service Delivery Reform	Health services are developed and delivered around the people and their needs and expectations.
Public Policy Reform	Pursue healthy public policies and strengthen national and transnational public health interventions.
Leadership Reform	Reflects inclusiveness, participatory, negotiation-based leadership.

Data from World Health Organization. (2008). *Primary health care: Now more than ever*. Geneva: Author. Retrieved from http://www.who.int/whr/2008/whr08_en.pdf

microbial diseases; (3) increasing access to essential, high-quality, effective, and affordable medical products; (4) addressing the social, economic, and environmental determinants of health as a means of reducing health inequalities within and between countries; (5) addressing the challenge of noncommunicable disease and mental health, violence, and injuries and disabilities; and (6) meeting health-related Millennium Development Goals (MDG): Unfinished agenda and future challenges (p. 27).

Ultimately, the WHO is dedicated to the achievement of health locally and globally through these six priorities via the development of multisectorial and coordinated efforts. The Twelfth Programme traces the origin of interest in social, economic, and environmental determinants of health to the Alma-Ata Declaration on primary health care.

Nursing and the WHO

From the very beginning, there was a conscious identification of the need for the actions of multiple individuals if the complex needs of any population were going to be addressed. This is seen in the Pholela Heath Centers and also seen in the Alma-Ata Declaration. Nursing is at the core a valuable asset to any PHC initiative. In fact, beginning in 1950, the Expert Committee on Nursing of the WHO issued their first report. This report discussed the essentiality of nursing in the process of meeting the needs of the population in the development of health programs and also discussed the quantity, quality, education, and appropriate use of nurses (WHO, 1950). A second report was published in 1952 and stated, "In studying its task the committee recognized that nursing is one element in services provided for the community by a health team, and that the role of nursing in any community depends on the health needs of the people of that community and on the availability of the services of other members of the team" (WHO, 1952, p. 3). Since these early years, many other reports have been published by the WHO Expert Committee on Nursing and may be retrieved from the WHO website (http://www.who.int/en/). A review of the WHO website and searching *nursing* yields information about many focus areas depicting nursing such as: (1) Nursing and Midwifery; (2) Nursing and Mental Health; (3) Nursing in WHO Regions such as Regions of the Americas–PAHO, South-East Asia Region, European Region, and Western Region; (4) Nursing and Patient Safety; as well as (5) a photo gallery titled Picturing Health: 35 Years of Photojournalism at WHO, which highlights photos featuring nursing. This may be viewed at the following link: http://www.who.int /features/2009/photoarchives/nursing/en/.

Reflections and Conclusions

The WHO emerged from the chaos of World War II, and the developing principles of PHC were articulated in the Alma-Ata Declaration. Rather than seeing these principles as either present or absent, they can be viewed as goals to be considered both in creating organizational structures and in how health care is delivered. There is widespread agreement that nursing is important in the process of the development of a system that exemplifies the principles of PHC. Nurses and the nursing profession are in position to be a major player in the four reforms outlined in *Primary Health Care Now More Than Ever* (WHO, 2008). Nurses are the *leaders* who have the vision and experience to lead the system toward PHC via *public policy* reform and *universal coverage* that will ultimately affect *service delivery* toward positive health outcomes. Nurses, however, will not engage in these major activities alone but with other leaders and community members. These challenges need to be embraced if the health of populations is to be improved and health disparities eliminated. The Robert Wood Johnson Foundation advocates a culture of health that brings together the many ideas of PHC. Nurses have an opportunity to participate in "weaving the threads of health" into the communities in which they serve (Lavizzo-Mourey, 2015).

> The health workforce is critical to PHC reforms. Significant investment is needed to empower health staff—from nurses to policy-makers— with the wherewithal to learn, adapt, be team players, and to combine biomedical and social perspectives, equity sensitivity and patient centeredness. Without investing in their mobilization, they can be an enormous source of resistance to change, anchored to past models that are convenient, reassuring, profitable and intellectually comfortable. If, however, they can be made to see and experience that primary health care produces stimulating and gratifying work, which is socially and economically rewarding, health workers may not only come on board but also become a militant vanguard. (WHO, 2008, p. 110)*

---

*Reprinted from World Health Organization. (2008). *Primary health care now more than ever.* Geneva: Author. Retrieved from http://www.who.int/whr/2008/whr08_en.pdf. Reprinted from The World Health Report 2008.

Chapter Activities

1. Take some time and reflect upon your own philosophy of nursing and health care. Once you have written this philosophy, move into small groups and share your work with one another.

2. Work in the same group and study the Alma-Ata Declaration. What aspects do you value most? What resonates with your own philosophy?

3. Think about a health care delivery system and discuss how nurses and nursing can integrate the principles of Alma-Ata into nursing practice.

References

Kark, S. L., & Cassel, J. (1952). The Pholela Health Centre: A progress report. *South African Medical Journal Suid-AfrikaanseTydskrif Vir Geneeskunde*, *26*(6), 101–104.

Kark, S. & Cassel, J. (2002). The Pholela Health Centre: A progress report. *American Journal of Public Health*, *92*(11), 1743–1747.

Lavizzo-Mourey, R. (2015). In it together—Building a culture of health. Retrieved from http://www.rwjf.org/en/about-rwjf/annual-reports/presidents-message-2015.html

Phillips, H. (2014). The return of the Pholela experiment: Medical history and primary health care in post-apartheid South Africa. *American Journal of Public Health*, *104*(10), 1872–1876.

Susser, M. (1993). A South African odyssey in community health: A memoir of the impact of the teachings of Sidney Kark. *American Journal of Public Health*, *83*(7), 1039–1042.

Tollman, S. M. (1994). The Pholela Health Centre—The origins of community-oriented primary health care (COPC). *South Africa Medical Journal (SAMJ)*, *84*(10), 653–658.

United Nations. (n.d.). *Charter of the United Nations*. Retrieved from http://www.un.org/en/documents/charter/intro.shtml

U.S. Department of Health and Human Services. (2015, M.ch 23). Determinants of health. Retrieved from http://www.healthypeople.gov/2020/about/foundation-health-measures/Determinants-of-Health#policymaking

World Health Organization. (n.d.). About WHO. Retrieved from http:www.who.int/about/en/

World Health Organization. (1950). *Technical report series No. 24-Expert committee on nursing*. Geneva: Author. Retrieved from http://apps.who.int/iris/bitstream/10665/39806/1/WHO_TRS_24.pdf?ua=1

World Health Organization. (1952). *Technical report #49. Expert committee on nursing. Second report*. http://apps.who.int/iris/bitstream/10665/39826/1/WHO_TRS_49.pdf?ua=1

World Health Organization. (1978). *Declaration of Alma-Ata*. Retrieved from http://www.who.int/publications/almaata_declaration_en.pdf?ua=1

World Health Organization. (2008). *Primary health care now more than ever*. Geneva: Author. Retrieved from http://www.who.int/whr/2008/whr08_en.pdf

World Health Organization. (2014). *Twelfth General Programme of Work 2014–2019: Not merely the absence of disease*. Retrieved from http://apps.who.int/iris/bitstream/10665/112792/1/GPW_2014-2019_eng.pdf?ua=1

World Health Organization. (n.d.). The Global Advisory Group on Nursing and Midwifery (GAGNM). Retrieved from http://www.who.int/hrh/nursing_midwifery/networks/en/

Yach, D., & Tollman, S. M. (1993). Public health initiatives in South Africa in the 1940s and 1950s: Lessons for a Post Apartheid era. *American Journal of Public Health*, *83*(7), 1043–1050.

Chapter **3**

Nursing's Role in Building a Culture of Health

Susan B. Hassmiller

Chapter Objectives

By the end of this chapter, you will be able to:

1. Identify the social determinants of health and explain how where people live, learn, work, and play affects their health.
2. Describe new nursing roles that are promoting health and keeping people healthier.
3. Explain how nurses can build a Culture of Health by taking a leadership role in addressing the social determinants of health within a primary health care perspective.

33

Introduction

The United States is unhealthy, resulting in poorer quality of life and lost productivity compared with other developed countries. On more than 100 measures, health in the United States lags behind other developed nations. People in 26 countries can expect to live longer than Americans (Braveman & Egerter, 2013). U.S. rankings for infant mortality have also fallen relative to other countries, from 18th in 1980 to 26th in 2006 (OECD, 2009). Yet the United States continues to spend more on medical care than any other country (**Figure 3-1**). The United States, in short, is getting poor value for its health care dollar. This chapter provides a way to address the disparities of health

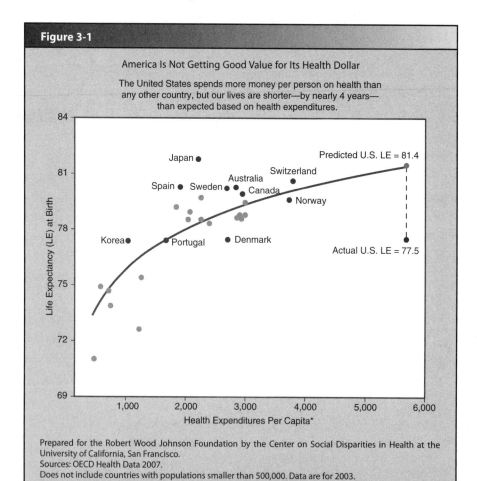

Figure 3-1

America Is Not Getting Good Value for Its Health Dollar

The United States spends more money per person on health than any other country, but our lives are shorter—by nearly 4 years—than expected based on health expenditures.

Prepared for the Robert Wood Johnson Foundation by the Center on Social Disparities in Health at the University of California, San Francisco.
Sources: OECD Health Data 2007.
Does not include countries with populations smaller than 500,000. Data are for 2003.
*Per capita health expenditures in 2003 U.S. dollars, purchasing power parity

Reproduced from Robert Wood Johnson Foundation Commission to Build a Healthier America. (2008). America Is Not Getting Good Value for Its Health Dollar. Retrieved from http://www.commissiononhealth .org/Charts.aspx care in the United States by changing the way we think in practice, moving toward the idea of primary health care, and developing a culture of health.

Health Disparities

Health varies substantially in the United States across states, cities, and regions and among social and economic groups, and many Americans are substantially less healthy than they could and should be (**Figure 3-2**; Egerter et al., 2009). The landmark Institute of Medicine report, *Unequal Treatment: Confronting Racial and Ethnic Disparities in Health Care* (Nelson, Smedley, & Stith, 2009), concluded that U.S. racial and ethnic minorities are less likely to receive routine medical procedures and experience a poorer quality of health services. The report found that a large body of research underscores the existence of disparities, defined as racial or ethnic differences in the quality of health care that are not due to access-related factors or clinical needs, preferences, or appropriateness of intervention (**Figure 3-3**). The mortality rate for Blacks has been 50% higher compared with Whites, and infant mortality for Blacks has been twice as high as that for Whites (National Center for Health Statistics, 2011; Satcher et al., 2005). The Department of Veterans Affairs, which offers patients similar access to care, has documented health disparities in its system, suggesting that disparities take root outside the formal health care system (Saha et al., 2008). Thomas LaVeist and his colleagues (2011) found that eliminating health disparities for minorities would have lowered direct medical care expenditures by $229.4 billion for the years 2003 through 2006.

The Social Determinants of Health

Where people live, learn, work, and play influences the choices Americans have for leading healthy lives. Our health-related behaviors are influenced by factors in our homes, schools, workplaces, and communities. Health disparities across income and education groups are present in many health conditions from the start of life to the end of life (Braveman, Cubbin, Egerter, Williams, & Pamuk, 2010). Each of us needs to take responsibility for making healthy choices about what we eat, how much we exercise, and whether to avoid smoking and other risky habits, but many Americans face obstacles that are too high to overcome on their own—even with great motivation. Black and Hispanic adults, for example, have less wealth, are more likely to have grown up in neighborhoods with fewer socioeconomic advantages, and are more likely to live in neighborhoods with concentrated poverty, insufficient housing, crime, and pollution and lack good schools, medical care, transportation, and jobs (Braveman et al. 2005; Williams & Jackson, 2005).

These factors—the nonmedical social, economic, political, or environmental factors that influence the distribution of health and illness in the population—are known as the social determinants of health (Gollust,

Figure 3-2

Across America, Differences in How Well and How Long We Live

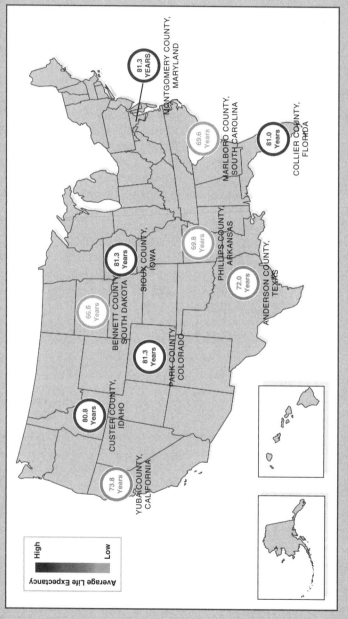

This map shows how life expectancy varies in different regions across the United States. The average life expectancy for people living in Bennett County, South Dakota, is 66.6 years. Just next door, people living in Sioux County, Iowa, can expect to live nearly 15 years longer.

Reproduced from Robert Wood Johnson Foundation Commission to Build a Healthier America. (2015). Across America, Differences in How Long and How Well We Live. Retrieved from http://www.commission onhealth.org/Charts.aspx

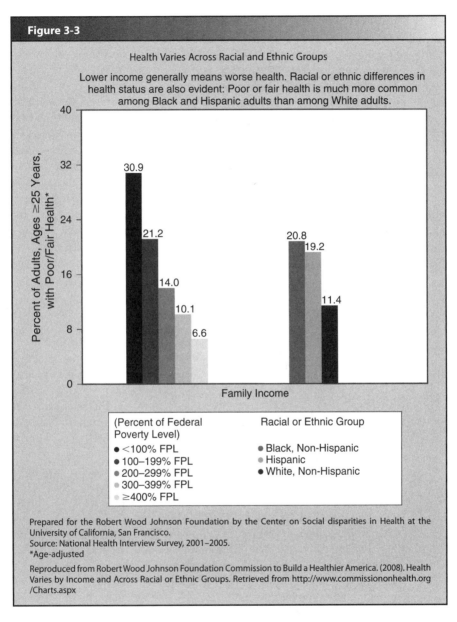

Figure 3-3

Health Varies Across Racial and Ethnic Groups

Lower income generally means worse health. Racial or ethnic differences in health status are also evident: Poor or fair health is much more common among Black and Hispanic adults than among White adults.

Family Income

(Percent of Federal Poverty Level)
- <100% FPL
- 100–199% FPL
- 200–299% FPL
- 300–399% FPL
- ≥400% FPL

Racial or Ethnic Group
- Black, Non-Hispanic
- Hispanic
- White, Non-Hispanic

Prepared for the Robert Wood Johnson Foundation by the Center on Social disparities in Health at the University of California, San Francisco.
Source: National Health Interview Survey, 2001–2005.
*Age-adjusted

Reproduced from Robert Wood Johnson Foundation Commission to Build a Healthier America. (2008). Health Varies by Income and Across Racial or Ethnic Groups. Retrieved from http://www.commissiononhealth.org/Charts.aspx

Lantz, & Ubel, 2009). Public health advocates have increasingly concluded that addressing the social determinants of health is necessary to improving health and health care in the United States and worldwide. The World Health Organization Commission on the Social Determinants of Health convened in 2006 to identify strategies that could improve health care around the world, reduce differences in health outcomes (Wilensky & Satcher, 2009), and subsequently describes efforts to tackle the social determinants of health as "fundamental" to its work (World Health Organization,

2015). The United States likewise is placing an increased emphasis on addressing the social determinants of health; they are included in *Healthy People 2020*, the government's 10-year goals and objectives for health promotion and disease prevention (*Healthy People 2020*, 2015).

The social determinants of health recognize that health is much more than health care. Virginia Commonwealth University's Steven Woolf (2009) points out that "perfecting health care is a half answer if the conditions that cause disease prevail" (p. 2). If we are going to address the root causes of disease, primary care professionals need to consider what happens when people leave the provider's office and return home. Do their homes, workplaces, leisure activities, communities, and neighborhoods support ongoing good health (Baum, Bégin, Houweling, & Taylor, 2009)? Efforts that simply inform or encourage individuals to change their behaviors, without also accounting for their physical and social environments, often do not reduce—and may even exacerbate—health inequalities (Glouberman, 2001). Health professionals, including nurses, can lower demand for care services by focusing on prevention and health promotion and considering the following factors.

Where People Live

Neighborhoods influence health in myriad ways, from the air and water quality that residents breathe, to the closeness of companies that produce or store hazardous substances, to whether homes expose residents to lead paint, mold, dust, or pest infestation (Giles-Corti & Donovan, 2002). Access to sidewalks, parks, and grocery stores can determine whether a family is able to exercise and eat healthy food (see **Figure 3-4**; Booth, Pinkston, & Poston, 2005). The availability and quality of schools, transportation, primary health care, and jobs can also influence health by shaping residents' opportunities to earn a living. Schools located in low-income neighborhoods are more likely to serve inexpensive processed foods and rely on income from vending machine contracts that promote soda and high-calorie snacks (Woolf, Dekker, Byrne, & Miller, 2011).

Neighborhoods where residents know and trust each other have been linked to lower homicide rates (Morenoff, Sampson, & Raudenbush, 2001), and less closely knit neighborhoods have been linked to anxiety and depression (Ross, 2000). A person's zip code at birth may be as important as his or her genetic code in predicting how well, and how long, he or she lives. For example, babies born and raised on the Red Line in the Washington, D.C., metro area can expect to live to be 84 years old. Conversely, babies born a few metro stops away in downtown Washington, D.C., can expect to live 7 years less.

Where People Learn

A person's education level affects a person's health. Adults without a high school diploma or equivalent are 3 times as likely as those with a college

Figure 3-4

Where We Live Affects Our Health

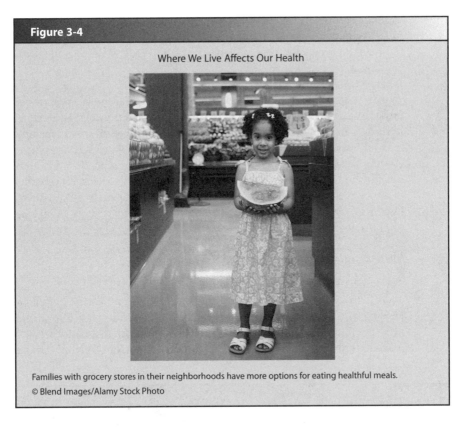

Families with grocery stores in their neighborhoods have more options for eating healthful meals.
© Blend Images/Alamy Stock Photo

education to die before age 65 (Heron et al., 2009). Men and women who have graduated from college can expect to live at least 5 years longer on average than adults who have not completed high school (Braveman & Egerter, 2008, 2013). Similarly, babies born to mothers who have completed less than 12 years of education are nearly twice as likely to die before their first birthday as babies born to mothers who have completed 16 or more years of schooling (Braveman & Egerter, 2008, 2013).

Where People Work

Poor Americans experience significantly worse health on average than wealthier Americans. In fact, U.S. adults living in poverty are more than 5 times as likely to report being in "fair" or "poor" health as adults with incomes at least 4 times the federal poverty level (Braveman & Egerter, 2008, 2013). People with lower incomes are more likely than people with higher incomes to lack a job, health insurance, and disposable income for medical expenses. Lower-income women are less likely to have access to onsite facilities for breastfeeding, which can promote health for babies. People with lower incomes may live in impoverished neighborhoods with limited employment opportunities and poorer quality schools. They often cannot afford to move elsewhere because traveling across town to find a job—or a better one—or to reach a grocery store or doctor may be difficult if public transportation is unavailable or costly (Woolf & Braveman, 2011).

Where People Play

The presence of sidewalks and playgrounds in neighborhoods, afterschool physical activity programs for children and youth, and the safety of a neighborhood can promote health by encouraging healthy behaviors and making it easier for people to adopt and maintain them (see **Figure 3-5**; Braveman, Egerter, & Mokenhaupt, 2011). Parents may want to send their children outside to play, but they may keep them in front of the television or computer because they fear for their safety. Other individuals may wish to bicycle or walk to work, but safe pedestrian routes or bicycle paths may be unavailable (Woolf & Braveman, 2011).

RWJF Commission to Build a Healthier America

The Robert Wood Johnson Foundation (RWJF), the nation's largest health and health care philanthropy, established the RWJF Commission to Build a Healthier America in 2008 to find ways to address the social determinants of health to improve our nation's health. The commission, a national nonpartisan group of leaders from the public and private sectors, issued

Figure 3-5

Where People Play

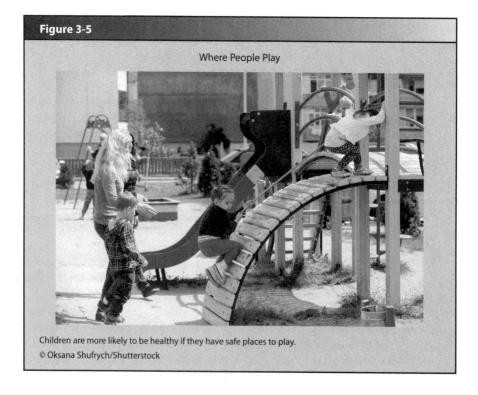

Children are more likely to be healthy if they have safe places to play.
© Oksana Shufrych/Shutterstock

10 sweeping recommendations aimed at improving the health of all Americans (see **Figure 3-6**; Miller, Simon, & Maleque, 2009). The commission's work led to a marked increase in collaboration among a wide variety of partners aimed at addressing the social determinants of health.

The commission reconvened in 2014 and issued a subsequent report. It found that to improve the health of all Americans we must:

- Invest in the foundations of lifelong physical and mental well-being in our youngest children;
- Create communities that foster health-promoting behaviors; and
- Broaden health care to promote health outside of the medical system (Robert Wood Johnson Foundation Commission to Build a Healthier America, 2014).

Building a Culture of Health

The commission's report coincided with RWJF's strategic shift to call on all Americans to help build a Culture of Health as the best way to improve health and health care in our nation. Building a Culture of Health is defined as shifting the values—and the actions—of this country so that health and

---

Figure 3-6

RWJF Commission to Build a Healthier America Recommendations, 2008

1. Fund and design WIC and SNAP (Food Stamps) programs to meet the needs of hungry families for nutritious food.
2. Create public–private partnerships to open and sustain full-service grocery stores in communities without access to healthful foods.
3. Feed children only healthy foods in schools.
4. Require all schools (K–12) to include time for all children to be physically active every day.
5. Become a smoke-free nation. Eliminating smoking remains one of the most important contributions to longer, healthier lives.
6. Ensure that all children have high-quality early developmental support (child care, education, and other services). This will require committing substantial additional resources to meet the early developmental needs particularly of children in low-income families.
7. Create "healthy community" demonstrations to evaluate the effects of a full complement of health-promoting policies and programs.
8. Develop a "health impact" rating for housing and infrastructure projects that reflects the projected effects on community health and provides incentives for projects that earn the rating.
9. Integrate safety and wellness into every aspect of community life.
10. Ensure that decision makers in all sectors have the evidence they need to build health into public and private policies and practices.

Reproduced from Robert Wood Johnson Foundation Commission to Build a Healthier America. (2009). Recommendations. Retrieved from http://www.commissiononhealth.org/Recommendations.aspx

healthy decisions become a part of everything Americans do. RWJF wants to enable all in our society to lead healthy lives, now and for generations to come. Too long our nation has defined being healthy as simply not being sick, and our health is often unduly and unequally influenced by income, education, ethnicity, and where a person lives.

The foundation wants to create a culture that empowers everyone to live the healthiest lives they can, even when they are dealing with chronic conditions or other challenges. RWJF imagines a health care system that couples treatment with care and considers the life needs of patients and caretakers, inside and outside the clinic. See **Figure 3-7** for the characteristics of a Culture of Health.

The Role of Nurses

Nurses are crucial to building a Culture of Health. At 3 million strong, nurses make up the largest segment of the health care workforce and spend the most time with people, families, and communities. Nurses are the glue that binds the system together, and they are vital to the successful transformation of health care. They provide holistic care across acute and community settings, which is increasingly important as care moves out of the hospital setting and into home and community settings. Nurses are at the center of many of the innovations we rely on to expand access, improve quality, and contain costs. And nurses with strong clinical and leadership skills can help to promote wellness, develop new models of care, and manage care coordination to help keep patients from returning to the hospital.

Figure 3-7

Characteristics of a Culture of Health in America

RWJF Vision for an American Culture of Health

1. Good health flourishes across geographic, demographic, and social sectors.
2. Being healthy and staying healthy is valued by our entire society.
3. Individuals and families have the means and the opportunity to make choices that lead to healthy lifestyles.
4. Business, government, individuals, and organizations work together to foster healthy communities and lifestyles.
5. Everyone has access to affordable, quality health care.
6. No one is excluded.
7. Health care is efficient and equitable.
8. The economy is less burdened by excessive and unwarranted health care spending.
9. The health of the population guides public and private decision-making.
10. Americans understand that we are all in this together.

Modified from Robert Wood Johnson Foundation. (2014). Building a Culture of Health: 2014 President's Message. Retrieved from http://www.rwjf.org/en/library/annual-reports/presidents-message-2014.html

In fact, nurses have a long history of promoting a Culture of Health. Florence Nightingale, the founder of modern nursing, expressed concern with the care of the sick poor in workhouses and workhouse infirmaries, including the quality of life in their homes and in the slums, which had high crime rates and rampant prostitution (see **Figure 3-8**). She sought to address the importance of preventing disease by teaching cleanliness and sanitation (Monteiro, 1985). Nightingale also recognized the importance of good child care to build health. "Money would be better spent in maintaining health in infancy and childhood than in building hospitals to alleviate or cure disease. It is much cheaper to promote health than to maintain people in sickness," she wrote in 1894 (Lundy, Janes, & Hartman, 2001).

Lillian Wald also devoted her life to building a Culture of Health after she was summoned in 1893 to the home of one of her immigrant students to care for the student's mother (**Figure 3-9**). She wrote of being guided through "evil smelling" streets, up slimy steps of a rear tenement into the

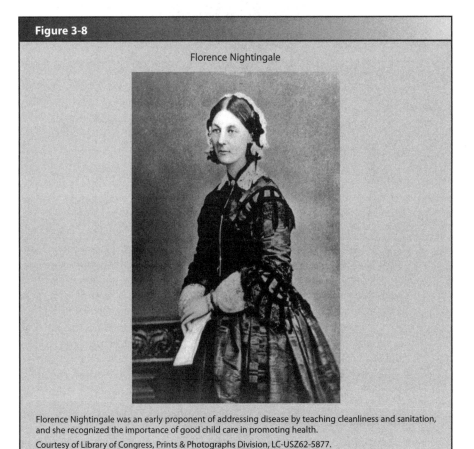

Figure 3-8

Florence Nightingale

Florence Nightingale was an early proponent of addressing disease by teaching cleanliness and sanitation, and she recognized the importance of good child care in promoting health.

Courtesy of Library of Congress, Prints & Photographs Division, LC-USZ62-5877.

Figure 3-9

Lillian Wald

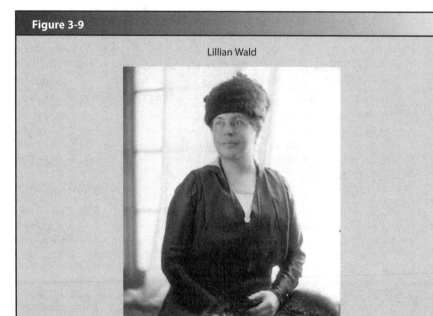

Wald was one of the first nurses to link sickness to a larger set of social problems. She incorporated health, industry, education, recreation, and housing into her work to improve life for residents of the lower-east-side of New York City.

Courtesy of Library of Congress, Prints & Photographs Division, photograph by Harris & Ewing, LC-DIG-hec-19537.

sickroom, where the "sick woman lay on a wretched, unclean bed, soiled with a hemorrhage two days old" (Wald, 1915). Wald recognized that the woman's sickness was part of a larger set of social problems, so she initiated a reform agenda that included health, industry, education, recreation, and housing. She established the Henry Street Settlement, which offered neighborhood residents health care, social services, and instruction in everything from English language to music. Nurses taught infant care to new mothers in their homes. They treated conditions that had previously kept children from entering the classroom. They offered cooking, sewing, music, and dance classes, and they established the city's first municipal playground (Buhler-Wilkerson, 1993).

Nurses have continued to improve health by addressing the factors that affect where people live, learn, work, and play ever since.

The Affordable Care Act

Passage of the Patient Protection and Affordable Care Act (ACA) in 2010 gives nurses new opportunities to deliver care (Hassmiller, 2010) and to help build a Culture of Health. With millions of Americans signing up for health insurance—some for the first time—policy makers increasingly are turning to more nurse practitioners and physician assistants to help address the primary care shortage. Compared to physicians, the number of nurse practitioners and physician assistants is expected to be much higher than the projected number of primary care doctors. The Association of American Medical Colleges (AAMC, 2010) estimates a shortfall of 45,000 primary care physicians by 2020. As a result, policy makers anticipate that nurse practitioners who practice with a primary health care perspective will help to alleviate the shortage under new models emphasizing team-based care, such as the patient-centered medical home and accountable care organizations (ACOs), which depend on a team of providers to deliver coordinated primary care across multiple settings. A national survey of primary care nurse practitioners and primary care physicians found that nurse practitioners are more likely to provide primary care in a wider range of settings, and provide proportionally more care to Medicaid recipients, racial and ethnic minorities, and uninsured populations (Buerhaus, DesRoches, Dittus, & Donelan, 2014).

In addition to increasing demand for primary care, the ACA includes provisions to promote wellness (Koh & Sebelius, 2010) and manage more carefully the high costs associated with care provided in hospitals (Berg & Dickow, 2014). Nurses bring traditional competencies such as care management and coordination, patient education, other public health interventions, and transitional care that will be especially valuable as the health system undergoes transformation to emphasize health promotion, illness prevention, risk reduction, and management rather than acute care. The landmark Institute of Medicine (IOM, 2011) report, *The Future of Nursing: Leading Change, Advancing Health*, stressed that nurses have an important contribution to make in "building a health care system that will meet the demand for safe, quality, patient-centered accessible and affordable care" (p. 21).

In many places throughout the United States, nurses are using their skills and competencies to address all of the factors that affect health. By seeking to improve where people live, learn, work, and play, nurses are on the frontlines of helping to build a Culture of Health.

Case Studies: Nurses Promoting a Culture of Health

Nurse-Family Partnership Program

Perhaps the best-known and well-researched example of nurses promoting a Culture of Health is the Nurse-Family Partnership (NFP) program, which takes a broad view of addressing the health and social needs of the individual and family. As part of the program, low-income first-time pregnant women receive home visits by nurses during their pregnancy and the first 2 years of their children's lives. During the home visits, nurses seek to improve prenatal care by ensuring the women receive needed treatment for pregnancy-related complications and reduce their use of cigarettes, alcohol, and illegal drugs. After the baby is born, the nurse focuses on improving the child's health by providing responsible and competent care during early childhood. The program also seeks to enhance educational and employment opportunities for the parents and plan future pregnancies (Olds, Sadler, & Kitzman, 2007).

The program has led to improvements in prenatal health-related behaviors; pregnancy outcomes, including reduced preterm delivery and lower rates of pregnancy-induced hypertension; lower rates of child abuse and neglect; lower rates of subsequent pregnancies; and higher employment rates of mothers (Olds, 2002). The program also resulted in improved school performance for the child. By age 19, youths whose mothers received visits from nurses nearly two decades earlier were 58% less likely to have been convicted of a crime (Olds et al., 2007).

The NFP had a high return on investment, with a net benefit to society of $17,180 (in 2003 dollars) per family served, which equates to a $2.88 return per dollar invested in NFP. In fact, the NFP program is being disseminated more broadly under the ACA.

Eleventh Street Family Health Services

The Eleventh Street Family Health Services Center of Drexel University in North Philadelphia prides itself on treating the whole person and creating community; it measures its success by the solid partnerships it shares with its community and the thousands of lives it has helped to change for the better. The nurse-managed health center started in 1996 when the College of Nursing entered into an agreement with the Philadelphia Housing Authority to address health issues of residents in Philadelphia's 11th Street corridor, where most of the 6,000 residents are Black, have low incomes, and are medically underserved. The neighborhood has the largest percentage of unemployed adults and families living in poverty, as well as the highest rate of diabetes within Philadelphia (Drexel University College of Nursing and Health Professions, n.d.).

Director Patricia Gerrity, a public health nurse and Associate Dean for Community Programs in the College of Nursing and Health Professions, stressed the importance of listening to the residents to earn their support. She placed a public health nurse at each of four housing developments in the neighborhood. The nurses responded to residents' immediate concerns, including the need for stop signs, animal control, food assistance, and training in CPR. By gaining trust of the residents, and making the residents' issues the defining issues, a long-term commitment was realized (Drexel University College of Nursing and Health Professions, n.d.).

Around the same time, her colleagues provided health screenings and managed chronic conditions. They went to local schools to teach children about healthy habits (RWJF, 2015). Community residents expressed interest for a health care center that they could access, regardless of their ability to pay.

In 1998 the health center opened, and in 2002, it gained status as a federally qualified health center. Nurse practitioners and social workers comprise teams that are enhanced as needed by physicians, nutritionists, and others. The center, which has 53 staff members, offers primary care, dental care, behavioral health care, physical therapy, and a vast array of community programs (**Figure 3-10**). The building includes a fitness center with a full-time personal trainer and a teaching kitchen where cooking classes take place. A community garden enables clients to grow fresh produce. Staff members work with local schools on public art projects, and nurses visit people at home to help them manage complex chronic conditions (RWJF, 2015).

Eleventh Street Family Health Services is an example of one of the more than 250 nurse-managed health clinics across the United States. These clinics, many of which are associated with schools of nursing, serve more than 2.5 million people and have emphasized the importance of addressing

Figure 3-10

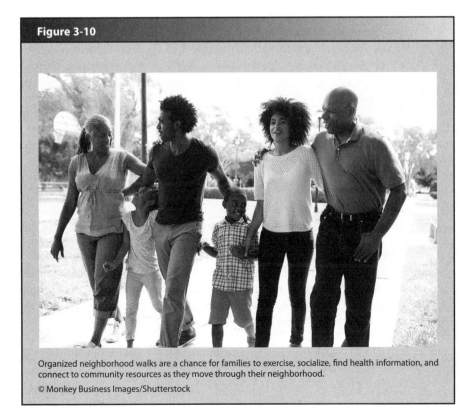

Organized neighborhood walks are a chance for families to exercise, socialize, find health information, and connect to community resources as they move through their neighborhood.

© Monkey Business Images/Shutterstock

the underlying factors that affect health. They offer accessible, affordable, quality health care and health services to underserved populations while also giving nursing and nurse practitioner students hands-on experience. Nurse-managed health clinics work closely with social workers to link their clients with other social service providers, and they build community by bringing health care to people in a neighborhood.

Transitional Care Model

Building a Culture of Health encompasses creating a culture that empowers every person to live the healthiest life, even when the person is dealing with chronic conditions or other challenges. Approximately 20% of hospitalized Medicare beneficiaries are readmitted within 30 days of leaving the hospital, and 34% return within 90 days, at an estimated cost in 2004 of $17.4 billion of the $102.6 billion in hospital payments from Medicare (Jencks, Williams, & Coleman, 2009). Enabling these people to stay safe in their homes and communities would go a long way toward reducing health care costs and promoting a Culture of Health. It would also benefit their family caregivers, who often have to take time off from work and suffer emotional distress and physical ailments from caring for loved ones (Reinhard, Levine, & Samis, 2012).

One nurse-led model that has overwhelmingly helped frail people to better manage their health is the Transitional Care Model. An advanced-practice registered nurse (APRN) meets with the patient and family caregivers when a patient is hospitalized to devise a plan for managing chronic illnesses. The APRN assists the patient and family in setting goals during the hospitalization, identifies the factors contributing to the patient's hospitalization, designs a care plan that addresses them, and coordinates the various care providers and services. Within the next 2 days, the nurse visits the patient at home and provides telephone and in-person support as often as necessary for up to 3 months. The nurse assesses, counsels, and accompanies the patient to medical appointments to help patients and their family caregivers learn the early signs of a problem that could require immediate help and to better manage the patient's health. The nurse also ensures that a primary care provider is assigned to the patient—as well as the requisite specialists—to keep track of everything affecting the patient (Naylor et al., 2004). The evidence overwhelmingly demonstrates the benefits of the Transitional Care Model. Three randomized controlled clinical trials of Medicare beneficiaries with more than one chronic illness showed that use of the Transitional Care Model lengthened the period between hospital discharge and readmission or death and resulted in fewer rehospitalizations (Naylor et al., 1994, 2004).

The University of Pennsylvania Health System has adopted the Transitional Care Model, and more than 24 health systems and communities are using parts of the model. As with the Nurse-Family Partnership, the ACA contains provisions that will support expansion of the Transitional Care Model.

Public Health Nursing

Building a Culture of Health will require an emphasis on population health and prevention, opening up a critical role for the nation's 34,500 nurses who work in state and local public health departments (University of Michigan, 2013). Public health nurses serve populations and can play a clear role in engaging communities around health, especially where people live, learn, work, and play. They can contribute to improving population-based health outcomes by offering reliable information on health and safety, and helping to promote early detection of common diseases (Hassmiller, 2014). Public health nurses also protect the public through infection control, emergency response, and health promotion initiatives (RWJF, 2015). In short, public health nurses address the root causes of problems. They use epidemiology and research to develop and test interventions that address poverty, housing, education, racism, adverse childhood experiences, and access to quality health care. A public health nurse could work with a group of neighborhood residents to secure space for a community garden and resources to plant and maintain the garden. He or she could organize a park cleaning event in a low-income neighborhood, or speak at the local planning commission about how safe sidewalks and open spaces promote healthy living. A public health nurse might also help new parents find resources for a child with special needs (Storey, 2013).

A great example of public health nurses working to build a Culture of Health is the Library Nurse Program, a join initiative between the public health department and the public library in Pima County, Arizona (see **Figure 3-11**). A team of public health nurses visits the city's 17 libraries to promote wellness and improve patrons' physical and mental health.

"Because they are perceived as safe and welcoming, public libraries have become shelters for people in need, the mentally ill, battered women, latchkey kids, and new immigrants," says Kathleen Malkin, division manager for Public Health Nursing Services at the Pima County Health Department, "so it makes sense to offer health services in this non-traditional setting" (RWJF, 2015, p. 6). Nurses tour the libraries with stethoscopes around their necks, talk with patrons, and offer health education. Though the program is available to everyone, it specifically targets people with mental health and social service needs. The areas of largest concern include malnutrition and poorly managed acute and chronic diseases. The public health nurses often connect patrons to social services to avoid crises. In the program's first month, behavior incidents were managed better, and the library made fewer nonmedical 911 calls (RWJF, 2015).

The Future of Nursing: Leading Change, Advancing Health

These examples represent nursing at its best and showcase the possibilities of nursing working in a new era of health and health care. However, the IOM

Figure 3-11

Public Health Nurse Making Rounds in a Library in Pima County, Arizona

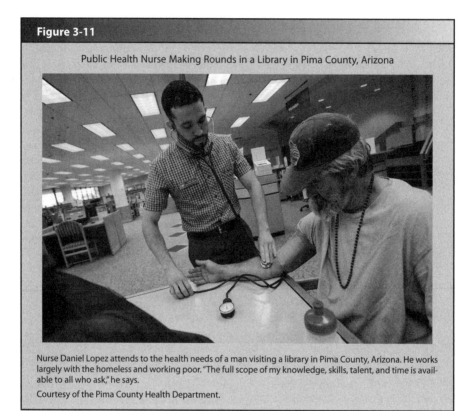

Nurse Daniel Lopez attends to the health needs of a man visiting a library in Pima County, Arizona. He works largely with the homeless and working poor. "The full scope of my knowledge, skills, talent, and time is available to all who ask," he says.

Courtesy of the Pima County Health Department.

(2011) report on the future of nursing recognizes that many more nurses will "require more education and preparation to adopt new roles quickly in response to rapidly changing health care settings and an evolving health care system" (p. 4). As a result, the IOM report issued sweeping recommendations to improve the health of the U.S. population through the contributions that nurses can make to the delivery of care (**Figure 3-12**).

The Robert Wood Johnson Foundation believed these recommendations were too important to sit on a shelf, so in 2010 it partnered with AARP, the nation's largest consumer organization, to start a national Campaign for Action to advance the IOM recommendations. The campaign works at both the national level and in the states, engaging with consumers, nurses, other clinicians, insurers, health care systems, employers, educators, funders, and policy makers—all the stakeholders who need to be involved in system change—to advance the IOM's recommendations.

The campaign has established Action Coalitions in all 50 states and the District of Columbia to pave the way for needed changes at the state level. As of January 2015, Action Coalitions collected a total of $11 million in

Figure 3-12

IOM Recommendations on the Future of Nursing

1. Remove scope-of-practice barriers.
2. Expand opportunities for nurses to lead and diffuse collaborative improvement efforts.
3. Implement nurse residency programs.
4. Increase the proportion of nurses with a baccalaureate degree to 80% by 2020.
5. Double the number of nurses with a doctorate by 2020.
6. Ensure that nurses engage in lifelong learning.
7. Prepare and enable nurses to lead change to advance health.
8. Build an infrastructure for the collection and analysis of interprofessional health care workforce data.

Republished with permission of The National Academies Press, from IOM (Institute of Medicine) 2011. *The Future of Nursing: Leading Change, Advancing Health*, pp. 9–14. Washington, DC: The National Academies Press. Permission conveyed through Copyright Clearance Center, Inc. https://nursing.unc.edu/files/2013/12/Future-Nursing-Report-IOM.pdf

funding from more than 800 organizations and individuals. Their members include a wide range of health care providers, consumer advocates, policy makers, business, academic, and philanthropic leaders. The campaign's vision is for everyone in America to live a healthier life, supported by a system in which nurses are essential partners in providing care and promoting health.

The campaign seeks to strengthen nursing education, remove scope-of-practice barriers, promote nursing leadership, foster interprofessional collaboration, and promote workforce diversity.

Nursing Education

The campaign strives to advance the IOM recommendation that 80% of the nursing workforce attain a bachelor's degree in nursing or higher by 2020; in 2010, when the report was released, 49% did so (according to data compiled by the American Community Survey Public Use Microdata Sample; Hassmiller & Reinhard, 2015). The campaign also wants to double the number of nurses with doctorates by 2020.

Rationale. Strengthening nursing education is crucial if more nurses are to take on more complex roles in our evolving health system. Nurses are needed to coordinate care for different types of patients; manage transitions across acute, ambulatory, and community settings; engage and educate patients and families; perform outreach and population health management; and connect patients with community-based services. Nurses need to have the competencies required to practice in the community, home, and public health settings.

In addition, nurses are needed to address the primary care shortage and the faculty shortage. Millions of new Americans now have health insurance through the ACA, and the United States is already struggling to provide primary care. Nurse practitioners can help to fill these roles. More nurses with doctorates are needed to teach the next generation and to design health care delivery innovations. In 2011, nursing schools turned away more than 75,000 qualified candidates, primarily because of a lack of school resources and faculty available to teach them (American Association of Colleges of Nursing [AACN], 2015b).

Progress made. The Action Coalitions have set out to advance nursing education by encouraging strong partnerships between community colleges and 4-year universities to make it easier for nurses to continue their education and earn advanced degrees. In 2014, the campaign showed that the number of nurses with a baccalaureate degree increased to 51%, and there was a 10% rise in the number of nurses with bachelor's degrees, from 1.37 million to 1.52 million. More nurses are enrolling in bachelor's programs, according to the American Association of Colleges of Nursing, and the number of enrollees in RN-to-BSN programs is expanding (Hassmiller & Reinhard, 2015).

Even more exciting, the number of nurses with doctoral degrees has increased substantially. In 2010, only 1% of the nation's 3 million nurses had doctoral degrees (IOM, 2011). From 2010 to 2013, the number of nurses enrolled in doctoral programs jumped 70%, from 11,645 to 19,828. The majority of this growth took place in the doctoral of nursing practice (DNP) programs, but enrollment in research-oriented PhD programs has also grown: in 2013, 5,140 students were enrolled in these programs, up from 4,611 in 2010 (Hassmiller & Reinhard, 2015).

Scope-of-Practice Barriers

Primary care in the United States is struggling to meet demand. Staffing shortages are expected to get worse as millions of newly insured Americans seek care, the population continues to age, and people grapple with more chronic disease. This is particularly true in underserved, rural, and minority communities. Nurse practitioners provide an immediate and cost-effective solution to this problem, enabling physicians to direct their energy to caring for people with complex medical conditions.

However, outdated barriers in many states prevent APRNs from expanding access to care (see **Figure 3-13**). Opponents of lifting restrictions on APRN practice contend that doing so will compromise quality of care and safety. However, the IOM (2011) report found no evidence that care provided in states that require APRNs to work under a physician's authority is better than in states where APRNs have full practice authority.

Progress made. Before the Campaign for Action began in late 2010, only 13 states and the District of Columbia allowed nurse practitioners to provide care to the full extent of their education and training. In the campaign's first

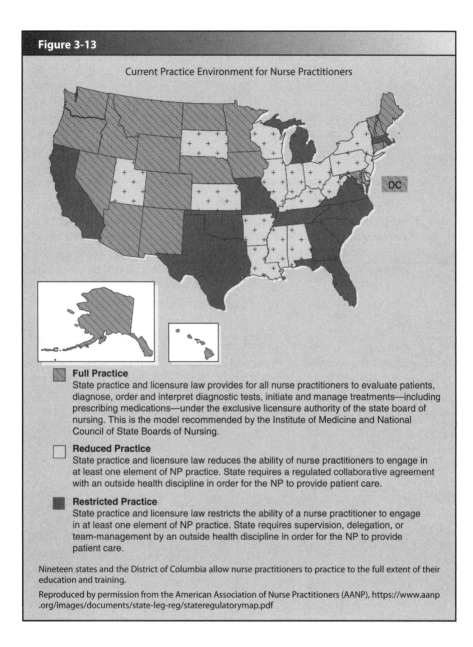

Figure 3-13

Current Practice Environment for Nurse Practitioners

Full Practice
State practice and licensure law provides for all nurse practitioners to evaluate patients, diagnose, order and interpret diagnostic tests, initiate and manage treatments—including prescribing medications—under the exclusive licensure authority of the state board of nursing. This is the model recommended by the Institute of Medicine and National Council of State Boards of Nursing.

Reduced Practice
State practice and licensure law reduces the ability of nurse practitioners to engage in at least one element of NP practice. State requires a regulated collaborative agreement with an outside health discipline in order for the NP to provide patient care.

Restricted Practice
State practice and licensure law restricts the ability of a nurse practitioner to engage in at least one element of NP practice. State requires supervision, delegation, or team-management by an outside health discipline in order for the NP to provide patient care.

Nineteen states and the District of Columbia allow nurse practitioners to practice to the full extent of their education and training.

Reproduced by permission from the American Association of Nurse Practitioners (AANP), https://www.aanp .org/images/documents/state-leg-reg/stateregulatorymap.pdf

4 years, 7 states (Connecticut, Kentucky, Minnesota, Nevada, North Dakota, Rhode Island, and Vermont) removed statutory barriers to give nurse practitioners full practice and prescriptive authority, bringing the total to 19 states and the nation's capital. Several states have achieved incremental improvements as well (Hassmiller & Reinhard, 2015).

Nursing Leadership

Nursing is repeatedly ranked the nation's most trusted profession (Rifkin, 2014). Nurses make up the largest group of health professionals, and they spend the most time with people and their caregivers. They provide an important and unique point of view in decision-making, from the boardroom to our communities. They are vital to improving quality by supporting the transition of patients from hospital to home or community and reducing rehospitalizations and medical errors. However, the IOM (2011) report pointed out that nurses seldom sit at leadership and policy-making tables and calls on nurses to take on increasing roles of responsibility in the health care system and society.

Progress made. Action Coalitions throughout the country are establishing programs that train nurses for leadership and board positions. They are also keeping track of open board positions and urging nurses to apply. The Campaign for Action has created the Nurses on Boards Coalition, a group of 21 national organizations that has pledged to place 10,000 nurses on boards by 2020.

Interprofessional Collaboration

As the case studies demonstrated, the future of health care will occur in teams, but it is difficult for professions to work well together if they have limited training and experience in schools. The IOM report called for an end to "educational silos" in which students from one profession are educated separately from other fields. In the 2013–2014 school year, of the 10 nursing schools with graduate health professional schools that were surveyed, 9 required at least one interprofessional course or activity—compared with 4 during the 2010–2011 school year (Hassmiller & Reinhard, 2015).

Workforce Diversity

The nursing workforce historically has been predominately White and female, and remains so today. More than one third of the U.S. population is part of a racial or ethnic minority according to the 2010 census (United States Census Bureau, n.d.), yet nurses from minority backgrounds represent only 19% of the registered nurse workforce, and men comprise 9.6% of all RNs (AACN, 2015). By 2043, minority populations will make up a majority of our population (United States Census Bureau, n.d.). Our profession should reflect the people we serve, and all nurses should be trained to deliver culturally competent services in all settings (**Figure 3-14**).

Progress made. The number of minority nurses in the workforce is gradually rising, and so is the share of the nursing workforce that they represent. Approximately 24% of the nursing workforce self-identified as minorities in 2010; that number is closer to 25% in 2012. Data collection is improving too. In 2011, 34 states collected race and ethnicity data on their nursing workforce; in 2013, 45 states did (Hassmiller & Reinhard, 2015).

Figure 3-14

Strengthening Workforce Diversity

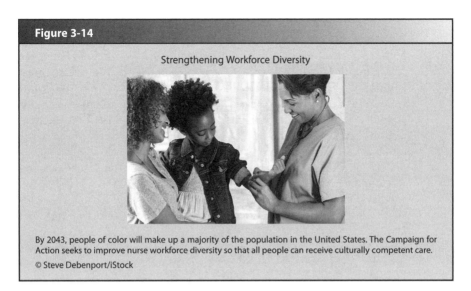

By 2043, people of color will make up a majority of the population in the United States. The Campaign for Action seeks to improve nurse workforce diversity so that all people can receive culturally competent care.

© Steve Debenport/iStock

Call to Action: The Future of Nursing and You

The Campaign for Action is making substantial progress in preparing the nursing workforce to take on new roles in the health system and to help build a Culture of Health that enables all in our society to lead healthier lives—but much more needs to be done. It will take all of us—health professionals, hospitals and health systems, policy makers, consumer advocates, payers, consumers, businesses, think tanks, long-term care, foundations, and everyone who cares about health care—to make this work. It will also take students.

You can help to build a Culture of Health by continuing your education no matter what your basic degree will be. Consider becoming nurse faculty and teaching the next generation of nursing students or becoming advanced practice registered nurses or public health nurses. You can take on greater roles in primary care to ensure that the Americans who gain access to health insurance under the ACA are able to see a practitioner when they need one and to receive routine preventive care. You can provide care coordination and chronic care management, as well as work in public health and community care.

If you choose to work at the bedside, you need to understand every aspect of your patient's very complex needs. You will need to pursue lifelong learning, as well as an advanced degree. Because of the constant changes in the health care system and patient demographics, an entry level degree is your entry point. It is up to you to stay current through continuous learning—you owe it to the people, families, and communities you serve to provide the most up-to-date care.

Pursue leadership as you embark on your career. Leadership needs to happen at every level. Speak up at your workplace if you have an idea for improving health. Seek out committees and consider volunteering in the community to broaden your experience. Volunteering also offers a great addition to any resume, especially if you are seeking your first job. Know your areas of expertise and develop your skill set. Strive to serve on boards as your career progresses and enter policy debates. Join professional associations, and volunteer with the Campaign for Action. Go to www.campaignforaction.org to sign up and get involved.

If you choose to get an advanced degree and pursue leadership, you will join the many nurses who are helping to build a Culture of Health. You will have opportunities to address health disparities and make it easier for all people to lead healthier lives, no matter where they live, learn, work, and play. According to Linda Reutter and Kaysi Eastlick Kushner (2010, p. 5), Cathy Crowe, a Toronto street nurse who advocates for the homeless, has summed up nursing's legacy well: "Throughout our history, it has been nurses who, after witnessing injustices, spoke out. They responded with words, with research, with action, with the development of programs, with legal action, and with new policy proposals." You are called to do the same: to help build a Culture of Health to enable all to lead healthier lives, now and for generations to come.

Chapter Activities

1. What are the social determinants of health, and how do they affect a person's health throughout the life span?

2. How can the nursing field use a primary health care perspective to address the social determinants of health?

3. In what ways do you see primary health care supporting a Culture of Health?

References

American Association of Colleges of Nursing. (March 16, 2015). Fact sheet: Enhancing diversity and the nursing workforce. Retrieved from http://www.aacn.nche.edu/media-relations/diversityFS.pdf

American Association of Colleges of Nursing. (2015b). *New AACN Data Show an Enrollment Surge in Baccalaureate and Graduate Programs Amid Calls for MoreHighly Educated Nurses.* Retrieved from http://www.aacn.nche.edu/news/articles/2012/enrollment-data

Association of American Medical Colleges Center for Workforce Studies. (2010). *Physician shortages to worsen without increases in residency training.* Retrieved from https://kaiserhealthnews.files.wordpress.com/2014/04/physician_shortages_to_worsen_without_increases_in_residency_tr.pdf

Baum, F. E., Bégin, M., Houweling, T. A., & Taylor, S. (2009). Changes not for the fainthearted: Reorienting health care systems toward health equity through action on the social determinants of health. *American Journal of Public Health,* 99(11), 1967–1974. Retrieved from http://www.ncbi.nlm.nih.gov/pmc/articles/PMC2759791/

Berg, J. G., & Dickow, M. (2014). Nurse role exploration project: The Affordable Care Act and new nursing roles. *Nurse Leader, 12*(5), 40–44.

Booth, K. M., Pinkston, M. M., & Poston, W. S. (2005). Obesity and the built environment. *Journal of the American Dietetic Association, 105,* 1110–1117.

Braveman, P. A., Cubbin, C., Egerter, S., Chideya, K., Marchi, K. S., Metzler, M., & Posner, S. (2005). Socioeconomic status in health research: One size does not fit all. *Journal of American Medical Association, 294*(22), 2879–2888.

Braveman, P. A., Cubbin, C., Egerter, S., Williams, D. R., & Pamuk, E. (2010). Socioeconomic disparities in health in the U.S.: What the patterns tell us. *American Journal of Public Health, 100*(S1), S186–S196.

Braveman, P., & Egerter, S. (2008). *Overcoming obstacles to health* (Report from the Robert Wood Johnson Foundation to the Commission to Build a Healthier America). Princeton, NJ: Robert Wood Johnson Foundation.

Braveman, P., & Egerter, S. (2013). *Overcoming obstacles to health in 2013 and beyond.* Princeton, NJ: Robert Wood Johnson Foundation.

Braveman, P. A., Egerter, S. A., & Mokenhaupt, R. E. (2011). Broadening the focus: The need to address the social determinants of health. *American Journal of Preventive Medicine, 40*(1), S4–S18.

Buerhaus, P. I., DesRoches, C. M., Dittus, R., & Donelan, K. (2014). Practice characteristics of primary care nurse practitioners and physicians. *Nursing Outlook, 63*(2), 144–153. doi: http://dx.doi.org/10.1016/j.outlook.2014.08.008

Buhler-Wilkerson, K. (1993). Bringing care to the people: Lillian Wald's legacy to public health nursing. *American Journal of Public Health, 83*(12), 1778–1786.

Drexel University College of Nursing and Health Professions (N.D.) Stephen and Sandra Sheller 11th Street Family Health Services., Retrieved from http://drexel.edu/cnhp/practices/11th-street/

Egerter, S., Braveman, P., Cubbin C., Dekker, M., Sadegh-Bobar, T., An, J., & Grossman-Kahn, R. (2009). *Reaching America's health potential: A state-by-state look at adult health.* Washington, DC: Robert Wood Johnson Foundation Commission to Build a Healthier America.

Giles-Corti, B., & Donovan, R. J. (2002). The relative influence of individual, social and physical environment determinants of physical activity. *Social Science and Medicine, 54*, 1793–1812.

Glouberman, S. (2001). *Towards a new perspective on health policy* (CPRN Study No. H-30). Ottawa ON: Canadian Policy Research Networks Inc.

Gollust, S. E., Lantz, P. M., & Ubel, P. A. (2009). The polarizing effect of news media messages about the social determinants of health. *American Journal of Public Health, 99*(12), 2160. Retrieved from http://www.ncbi.nlm.nih.gov/pmc/articles/PMC2775784/

Hassmiller, S. (2010). Nursing's role in healthcare reform. *American Nurse Today, 5*(9), 68–69.

Hassmiller, S. B. (2014). Leveraging public health nursing to build a culture of health. *American Journal of Preventive Medicine, 47*(5 Suppl 3), S391–S392.

Hassmiller, S. B., & Reinhard, S. C. (2015). A bold new vision for America's health care system. *American Journal of Nursing, 115*(2), 49–55.

Healthy People 2020. (2015). *Social determinants.* Retrieved from http://www.healthypeople.gov/2020/leading-health-indicators/2020-lhi-topics/Social-Determinants

Heron, M., Hoyert, D. L., Murphy, S. L., Xu, J. Q., Kochanek, K. D., & Tejada-Vera, B. (2009). Deaths: Final data for 2006. *National Vital Statistics Report, 57*(14), 1–134.

Institute of Medicine. (2011). *The future of nursing: Leading change, advancing health.* Washington, DC: National Academies Press.

Jencks, S. F., Williams, M. V., & Coleman, E. A. (2009). Rehospitalizations among patients in the Medicare fee-for-service program. *New England Journal of Medicine, 360*(14), 1418–1428.

Koh, H. K., & Sebelius, K. G. (2010). Promoting prevention through the Affordable Care Act. *New England Journal of Medicine, 363*(14), 1296–1299.

LaVeist, T. A., Gaskin, D. J., & Richard, R. (2011). Estimating the economic burden of racial health inequalities in the United States. *International Journal of Health Services, 41*, 231–238.

Lundy, K. S., Janes, S., & Hartman, S. (2001). Opening the door to health care in the community. In K. S. Lunday & S. Janes (Eds.), *Community health nursing: Caring for the public's health* (pp. 4–29). Sudbury, MA: Jones and Bartlett.

Miller, W., Simon, P., & Maleque, S. (2009). *Beyond healthcare: New directions to a healthier America* (Report from Robert Wood Johnson Foundation to Build a Healthier America). Washington, DC: Robert Wood Johnson Foundation.

Monteiro, L. A. (1985). Florence Nightingale on public health nursing. *American Journal of Public Health, 75*(2), 181–186.

Morenoff, J. D., Sampson, R. J., & Raudenbush, S. W. (2001). Neighborhood inequality, collective efficacy, and the spatial dynamics of urban violence. *Criminology, 39*, 517–558.

National Center for Health Statistics. (2011). *Health, United States, 2010: With special feature on death and dying* (DHHS Pub No. 2011-1232). Hyattsville, MD: Author. Retrieved from http://www.cdc.gov/nchs/data/hus/hus10_InBrief.pdf

Naylor, M., Brooten, D., Jones, R., Lavizzo-Mourey, R., Mezey, M., & Pauly, M. (1994). Comprehensive discharge planning for the hospitalized elderly: A randomized clinical trial. *Annals of Internal Medicine, 120*(12), 999–1006.

Naylor, M. D., Brooten, D. A., Campbell, R. L., Maislin, G., McCauley, K. M., & Schwartz, J. S. (2004). Transitional care of older adults hospitalized with heart failure: A randomized, controlled trial. *Journal of the American Geriatrics Society, 52*(5), 675–684.

Nelson, A. R., Smedley, B. D., & Stith, A. Y. (Eds.). (2009). *Unequal treatment: Confronting racial and ethnic disparities in health care* (with CD, Vol. 1). Washington, DC: National Academies Press.

Olds, D. L. (2002). Prenatal and infancy home visiting by nurses: From randomized trials to community replications. *Prevention Science, 3*(3), 153–172.

Olds, D., Sadler, L. S., Kitzman, H. (2007). Programs for parents of infants and toddlers: Recent evidence from randomized trials. *Journal of Child Psychology and Psychiatry, 48*, 355–391.

Organization for Economic Co-operation and Development, Directorate for Employment, Labour and Social Affairs. (2009). *OECD Health data: Frequently requested data.* Retrieved from http://www.oecd.org/els/

Reinhard, S. C., Levine, C., & Samis, S. (2012). *Home alone: Family caregivers providing complex chronic care.* Washington, DC: AARP Public Policy Institute.

Reutter, L., & Kushner, K. E. (2010). Health equity through action on the social determinants of health: Taking up the challenge in nursing. *Nursing Inquiry, 17*(3), 269–280.

Riffkin, R. (2014). *Americans rank nurses highest on honesty, ethical standards.* Retrieved from http://www.gallup.com/poll/180260/americans-rate-nurses-highest-honesty-ethical-standards.aspx

Robert Wood Johnson Foundation. (2015, April). The value of nursing in building a culture of health (Part 1): Reaching beyond traditional care settings to promote health where people live, learn, and play. *Charting Nursing's Future.* Retrieved from http://www.rwjf.org/en/library/research/2015/04/the-value-of-nursing-in-building-a-culture-of-health--part-1-.html

Robert Wood Johnson Foundation Commission to Build a Healthier America. (2014). *Time to act: Investing in the health of our children and communities.* Retrieved from http://www.rwjf.org/en/library/research/2014/01/recommendations-from-the-rwjf-commission-to-build-a-healthier-am.html

Ross, C. E. (2000). Neighborhood disadvantage and adult depression. *Journal of Health Social Behavior, 41*, 177–187.

Saha, S., Freeman, M., Toure, J., Tippens, K. M., Weeks, C., & Ibrahim, S. (2008). Racial and ethnic disparities in the VA healthcare system: A systematic review. *Journal of General Internal Medicine, 23*(5), 654–671.

Satcher, D., Fryer, G. E., McCann, J., Troutman, A., Woolf, S. H., & Rust, G. (2005). What if we were equal? A comparison of the Black-White mortality gap in 1960 and 2000. *Health Affairs, 24*(2), 459–464. doi: 10/1377/hitaff.24.2.459

Storey, M. (2013, August 2). Are you considering a career in public health nursing? [Weblog post]. Retrieved from http://www.rwjf.org/en/culture-of-health/2013/08/are_you_considering.html

United States Census Bureau. (n.d.). 2010 census press release: 2010 census shows America's Diversity. Retrieved from http://www.census.gov/newsroom/releases/archives/2010_census/cb11-cn125.html

University of Michigan Center of Excellence in Public Health Workforce Studies. (2013). *Enumeration and characterization of the public health nurse workforce:*

Findings of the 2012 public health nurse workforce surveys. Ann Arbor, MI: University of Michigan.

Wald, L. D. (1915). *The house on Henry Street.* New York, NY: Henry Holt and Company.

Wilensky, G. R., & Satcher, D. (2009). Don't forget about the social determinants of health. *Health Affairs, 28*(2), w194–w198.

Williams, D. R., & Jackson, P. B. (2005). Social sources of racial disparities in health. *Health Affairs, 24*(2), 325–334.

Woolf, S. H. (2009). Social policy as health policy. *Journal of American Medical Association, 301*(11), 1166–1169.

Woolf, S. H., & Braveman, P. (2011). Where health disparities begin: The role of social and economic determinants and why current policies may make matters worse. *Health Affairs, 30*, 1852–1859. Retrieved from http://content .healthaffairs.org/content/30/10/1852.full

Woolf, S. H., Dekker, M. M., Byrne, F. R., & Miller, W. D. (2011). Citizen-centered health promotion: Building collaborations to facilitate healthy living. *American Journal of Preventive Medicine, 40*(1 Suppl 1), S38–S47. doi: 10.1016 /j.amepre.2010.009.025

World Health Organization. (2015). *Social determinants of health.* Retrieved from http://www.who.int/social_determinants/en/

Social Justice, Nursing Advocacy, and Health Inequities: A Primary Health Care Perspective

Selina Mohammed, Christine A. Stevens, Mabel Ezeonwu, and Cheryl L. Cooke

Chapter Objectives

By the end of this chapter, you will be able to:

1. Articulate the important role of nurses in social justice and advocacy.
2. Examine the function of social justice and advocacy in addressing health inequities.
3. Explore multilevel strategies for promoting social justice and rectifying health injustices.

Introduction

In 2007, Margaret Chan, director of the World Health Organization (WHO), emphasized the need for a renewal in primary health care as an essential approach to improving health (WHO, 2007). After this conference, the WHO (2008) published *Primary Health Care: Now More Than Ever*, which examined the 1978 Declaration of Alma-Ata and expounded on reforms essential to the renewal of primary health care: issues of social justice and health equity. This report structured the requisite primary health care reforms into four groups: universal coverage reforms, service delivery reforms, public policy reforms, and leadership reforms. An important function of this report was to clarify the role of health professionals in primary health care. Delineation of this role underscored the centrality of health care providers in achieving goals of social justice and health equity, and specifically called on nurses not only to consider the context of patient's lives but to advocate for social justice and health care rights (WHO, 2008).

In the United States, several organizations representing the interests of nurses and the advancement of the nursing profession support the WHO's charge that nurses serve as advocates for social justice. For example, the American Nurses Association (ANA, 2015) *Position Statements on Ethics and Human Rights* has standards that clearly declare nurses as being responsible for advocating for all individuals in areas of health and health care rights. The position statements examine the continuum of advocacy required by nurses to address issues of ethics and social justice and define the function of nursing advocacy in individual and societal realms. The ANA was directive in their charge to nursing education leaders and faculty that students need to develop competencies in ethics, advocacy, and human rights at the individual, community, and global level.

In an effort to guide and streamline the education curriculum standards for nurses at baccalaureate and graduate levels, the American Association of Colleges of Nursing (AACN), which serves as one of the "national voices" for nursing education, has written a series of *Essentials* documents that outline competency expectations for graduates at each educational level. Nursing schools use these *Essentials* to develop educational programs that adhere to the highest standards of the nursing profession and to ensure they meet accreditation guidelines (AACN, 2008, 2011). The *Essentials* have clearly stated that "advocating for social justice and for patients" is required in the education of all levels of nursing students in varying degrees (AACN, 1996, 2006, 2008, 2011).

Standards in *The Essentials of Baccalaureate for Professional Nursing Practice*, for example, note that social justice is fundamental to the discipline of nursing and require that all baccalaureate students develop skills to provide leadership in promoting advocacy, collaboration, and social justice (AACN, 2008). Advocacy for vulnerable populations in pursuit of social justice and the elimination of health disparities is recognized as a moral and ethical responsibility of a nurse. This requires an understanding of the implications of health care policies, specifically how they relate to issues of equity and social justice, and engagement in these processes. The *Essentials of Master's Education for Advanced Practice Nursing* stresses ethical decision-making in graduate content that includes

> provid[ing] students the opportunity to explore their values and analyze how these values shape their professional practice and influence their decisions, and to analyze systems of health care and determine how the values underpinning them influence the interventions and care delivered. (1996, p. 9)

Furthermore, in *The Essentials of Doctoral Education for Advanced Nursing Practice*, the AACN (2006) has broadened the focus and scope of nursing advocacy in the promotion of social justice for nurses at this educational level. Advanced practice nurses are not only expected to understand the influence of health care policies, they are expected to help design, implement, and advocate for ethical health care policies at institutional and societal levels that address issues of social justice and equity.

As evidenced by the ANA and the AACN, the role of advocating for social justice is clearly expected of nurses who function within the world of primary health care. Benner, Sutphen, and Day (2010) state that one of the true hallmarks of a nursing professional is "moral imagination," which allows us to quickly see ethical dilemmas and imagine how to change how we care for vulnerable people. As primary health care providers, nurses are called upon to use their moral imagination to move beyond the perceived limits of their profession and advocate for the rights of patients, communities, and global societies in the pursuit of social justice.

Defining Social Justice and Advocacy

To rise to the call of advocacy in pursuit of social justice, nurses must first understand fundamentally what social justice and advocacy mean. On the surface, defining these terms seems to be a straightforward task. However, the literature reveals that consistent conceptions of social justice and advocacy remain elusive (Grace & Willis, 2012; Reimer Kirkham & Anderson, 2010). It is important to recognize that the work of advocacy in social justice problematically invokes politics of inclusion and difference, Othering, and relations of power[1] (Canales, 2000; Drevdahl, 2013; Reimer et al., 2010). Here these concepts provide a foundation for explaining why social justice

---

[1] These concepts all involve power differentials in society that serve to privilege members of dominant society and marginalize others. As used in this sentence, these concepts refer to unequal power relationships between advocates and people who are advocated for, and calls into question who has the right to speak for whom.

and advocacy should be viewed as core functions in nursing, and how they are vital to eliminating health disparities and achieving health equity.

Discourse on social justice vary within and across disciplines and continually evolve in complexity (Boutain, 2004; Buettner-Schmidt & Lobo, 2012; Grace & Willis, 2012; Pauly, MacKinnon, & Varcoe, 2009; Reimer Kirkham & Browne, 2006; Thompson, 2014). Through an analysis of the meanings and effects of social justice presented within nursing literature, Thompson (2014) found similar lines of analysis among nurse scholars and represented a collective definition of social justice as follows:

> (a) interventions focused on social, political, economic, and environmental factors that systematically disadvantage individuals and groups; and (b) intervening in the effects of power, race, gender, and class where these and other structural relations intersect to create avoidable disparities and inequities in health for individuals, groups, or communities. (p. E18)

Social justice involves not only critiquing but also challenging and changing the status quo. It entails an individual and collective accountability to rectify injustices for the most vulnerable groups to achieve equitable burdens and benefits in society (Boutain, 2004; Mohammed, Cooke, Ezeonwu, & Stevens, 2014).

Complementary to social justice is the concept of advocacy. Advocacy has been defined as the act of arguing on behalf of a particular issue, idea, or people (Ingram, Sabo, Rothers, Wennerstrom, & de Zapien, 2008); pleading the case of another or championing a cause; and empowering those less able to present their views or needs, with the goal of giving them a voice so they can achieve their objectives (Allender, Rector, & Warner, 2010). Advocacy is also described as coordinating with and intervening in systems on clients' behalf, and, in turn, empowering clients to do the same by providing adequate and appropriate information for them to make needed changes (Chafey, Rhea, Shannon, & Spencer, 1998). When individuals engage in advocacy, they take a position on an issue and initiate actions in a deliberate attempt to influence private and public policy choices (Labonte, 1994). These individuals use their position to support, protect, or speak out for the rights and interests of another (Zolnierek, 2012).

It is evident from these definitions that advocacy is not a single act but rather a series of actions that health providers can perform to address injustices and pursue health equity. Nurses have an individual and a collective responsibility to be health advocates and to use their knowledge and expertise to advance the health of individuals, families, communities, and populations (ANA, 2015). Increasingly, nurses are being called upon to broaden the scope of how they see themselves function within their profession and to support, create, and advocate for social justice strategies and policies that promote population health. It is imperative to understand the importance of this call.

Social Justice and Advocacy: Why Nurses Must Be Involved

A focus on health disparities and how to eliminate them has established that many of the primary drivers of health stem from the context of our everyday living (Carey & Crammond, 2015). These living conditions are often demonstrative of societal injustices, which are related in particular to the social determinants of health. As a result, the phrase "health inequities" is increasingly used in discourses on nursing and health to signify a shift from the language of "health disparities," which at a basic level underscores the systematic health differences adversely affecting socially disadvantaged groups (Braveman, 2014; Braveman, Egerton, & Williams, 2011). Health inequities more explicitly captures the moral dimension and introduces a strong judgment of causality, linking identified health differences to social, political, and economic injustices that are deep-seated and seemingly natural in our society (Braveman et al., 2011; Falk-Rafael & Betker, 2012). As noted by Braveman (2014), measuring health inequities relies on the metric of health disparities, which in turn, is the metric for health equity.

According to *Healthy People 2020*, health equity is a desirable goal that requires continuous efforts to eliminate health disparities (U.S. Department of Health and Human Services [USDHHS], 2014). Reducing health inequities and improving the health of socially disadvantaged populations may be achieved by addressing the social determinants of health. These determinants of health include health care and access to health care, but they also include the social and material conditions in which people live, work, learn, and play (Robert Wood Johnson Foundation [RWJF], 2014). Since a range of social, political, economic, and environmental factors is responsible for the unequal and avoidable differences in health status within and between populations (USDHHS, 2014), nurses must be responsive to the diverse needs of the populations they care for and advocate for appropriate programs and policies that target social determinants of health.

Nurses are in a prime position to engage in social justice advocacy and to lead initiatives that aim to reduce health inequities for several reasons. Nurses often work intimately with members of vulnerable populations and, therefore, maintain a close proximity to health care consumers. The inside perspectives gathered from individual, family, and community interactions, as well as knowledge regarding health and the health care system, help position nurses to intervene on behalf of these groups (Falk-Rafael, 2005). In addition, nurses are trained to take a holistic approach, giving them a broad perspective from which to view health and illness. Nurses also constitute the largest segment of the nation's health workforce (Health Resources and Services and Administration [HRSA], 2010). As the most versatile and populous group of health professionals, nurses are key in promoting primary health care and influencing public policy that improves health for socially disadvantaged groups. Furthermore, the expanded care access to millions of people through the Patient Protection and Affordable Care Act

(ACA) amplifies nursing's leadership roles in primary health care. According to the USDHHS (2011), the triple aims of the ACA are to (1) improve the individual experience of health, (2) improve the health of populations, and (3) reduce per capita costs of care for populations. In addition to the two aims that are specific to population health, one of the ways the ACA promotes health care is through value-based care models and incentives (Luther & Hart, 2014). Together, these foci have the potential to stimulate forward thinking plans and policies from nurses that address social determinants of health.

The presence and visibility of nurses in almost every health care setting make them undeniably central to the success of primary health care and social justice initiatives. By working in multiple levels of society, nurses have the opportunity to effect change within and outside of their employment organizations (Thompson, 2014). Being an advocate for health is fundamental to what nurses do and an essential part of the moral and ethical obligation of a profession that burgeoned from the context of caring. Working to reduce health disparities and improve the health of vulnerable populations is also part of the core values and predisposition of nursing. However, directing these essences into macro-level actions and policies that target social structures that create and sustain population health inequities is an area where nursing, as a profession, needs to grow and gain proficiency.

Barriers to Nurses' Involvement

Although social justice engagement has historic cornerstone roots in public health nursing, the nursing profession has professed the need for social justice more than it has demonstrated its operationalization (Anderson et al., 2009; Buettner-Schmidt & Lobo, 2012). There are several reasons for this focal shift. The values of neoliberal individualism and capitalist market economies, which create structures that produce and sustain inequities, is one reason for this shift (Thompson, 2014). As a result, contemporary governments privilege "downstream" behavioral health promotion strategies, which aim to improve health by influencing individual lifestyle factors as opposed to driving "upstream" health policies that target the social determinants of health (Baum & Fisher, 2014). In this vein, health is viewed primarily as a product of genetics or lifestyle choices, and responsibility for health is ascribed to the individual rather than being viewed as a collective issue and a product of sociopolitical, economic, and environmental determinants.

The biomedical model, which is the predominant health care delivery system in the United States, also reinforces the notion of individualism by narrowly defining health as the absence of disease and directing the bulk of health care resources to medical services and crisis interventions (Baum & Fisher, 2014; Day, 2010). In this model, health is primarily seen to be a product of individual choice, and group differences in health are seen as the cumulative result of group members' choices (Levinson, as cited in Baum & Fisher, 2014). The separation of health from broader social and economic determinants debunks the concept of health as a collective issue, and it can lead to a misconception of why some groups of people bear a disproportionate amount of illness compared to other groups and sustain personal and institutional racialized discrimination (Mohammed, 2014).

Another reason that nurses have not been more involved in the operationalization of social justice is due to its obscurity in the discourse of nursing. On a personal level, some nurses may believe that it is irrelevant for their professional practice. For instance, nurses who practice in acute care settings may believe that social justice is important in public health nursing, but not pertinent to their own specialty (Thompson, 2014). In addition, nurses may subscribe to professional models that promote their roles as specialists versus contributors to the "democratization of health," where nurses help develop public capacities to rectify structures that disadvantage populations (Thompson, 2014). At the professional level, a critique of three national nursing documents produced by the ANA demonstrated that these materials present inconsistent and ambiguous conceptualizations of social justice, and fail to offer adequate frameworks for nurses to address broad systems that affect health (Bekemeier & Butterfield, 2005). How can nurses be expected to engage in social justice and advocacy to address health inequities when there is a lack of clarity surrounding these concepts and a dearth of best practice examples regarding how nurses can implement them?

Moving Forward

To address health inequities, nurses need to adopt a multidimensional and broader vision of health (beyond the absence of disease) and have the political will to make changes. An understanding of the effects of social determinants on health and a commitment to undertaking upstream actions that address social injustices has the potential to change individualistic notions of health to conceptualizations of health as a collective issue. Nurses can be involved in this transformation in several ways. For example, nurse educators can focus their curricula on emancipatory knowledge development to uncover processes that produce and sustain social injustices (Chinn & Kramer, 2008). Yanicki, Kehsner, and Reutter (2014) recommend a greater emphasis on social justice in education, coupled with an examination of the root causes of health inequities and identification of multilevel interventions for change. Examples of these kinds of curricula and how they are enacted in the classroom are available (Mohammed et al., 2014). In addition, nurse researchers can continue to make visible the links between health inequities and social injustices. Furthermore, scholarship that illustrates multidimensional approaches to social justice advocacy within different practice contexts can benefit nurses who may be struggling in their conceptualizations of how to intervene and target the social determinants of health (Yanicki et al., 2014).

Although there are numerous nursing interventions that attempt to change health behaviors, it is challenging to finding interventions with a multifaceted approach in which the intervention addresses the effects of sociopolitical, economic, and environmental determinants on health. To gain a deeper understanding of what it means to develop a meaningful social justice and advocacy practice, we offer an example of a nurse interventionist doing this type of work and a program that is focused on improving health by addressing social determinants that contribute to poorer health outcomes.

Case Example: Moving Together in Faith and Healing (Boutain, McNees, & MTFH Collaborative, 2013)

Lead Investigator: Dr. Doris Boutain, School of Nursing, University of Washington

Funder: Department of Health and Human Services, Seattle King County Public Health

Participants: Six local Baptist, AME, and Catholic Churches and Just Gardens in Central & South Seattle, and Greater King County, Seattle, WA

Addressing a long-standing social justice problem of poor access to high-quality, nutritious food in Seattle's Central District, Boutain (a registered nurse and educator) developed a partnership between local churches, the local public health department, and Just Gardens, a local not-for-profit whose mission includes safeguarding natural resources to build gardens and improve food stability in low-income areas. The goal of this program, Moving Together in Faith and Healing (MTFH), is to aid in childhood obesity prevention. The program was built around influential churches whose communities are primarily African American and Pacific Islanders, two populations that suffer from disparate rates of diabetes, hypertension, and heart disease. The churches are the center of the programs, and the MTFH team employs strategies to advance the churches' missions of faith and health by becoming institutions that also establish legacies centered on building and sustaining healthy communities through modeling healthy eating and active living environments. As a way to encourage sustainability and focus on the larger sociocultural environment, churches that participate in the program build expertise to guide other area churches and community leadership in developing food security programs in their areas. The long-term goals of the program include building a community that brings health, nutritious food, and healthy movement to all.

The gardens were so successful that the MTFH team arranged for a weekly "wholesale food market" in the summer of 2011 that served the community by bringing food grown in the gardens and food grown by smaller farms that have difficulty generating higher sales to be sold to residents of Seattle's Central District. In this way, the local churches are building capacity around health and nutrition; community members who are economically disenfranchised benefit from continued access to wholesome foods; and the local farming community has an additional venue to sell their produce, thereby allowing for financial stability and continued local farming efforts. The sustainability of this program lies in the ability of these churches to create yearly gardens that bring wholesome foods to a community where food insecurity and childhood obesity exist.

The MTHF program outcomes were focused on policy, systems, and environmental change, and findings from the evaluation of the MTHF were demonstrated in each of these areas (Boutain et al., 2013). Early changes were primarily environmental in nature and included removal of vending machines from churches, serving water at church events, and changing the order of when fruits and vegetables were served during church dinners. Policy and systems changes occurred in mid- and late-stages a year or more into the program. Examples of these include the churches creating policies and procedures to ensure lasting change and developing relationships with local grocery stores (that include a reduced cost for nutritious foods at church functions), building and sustaining community gardens, and constructing official budgets for health ministries. Ultimately, by sharing their successes and encouraging broader social changes, churches can work together to change neighborhood environments nationwide into places where faith and health opportunities are affordable and accessible to everyone (Boutain et al., 2013).

What made the Moving Together in Faith and Health project so successful? Part of their success was determined by critical and sustained involvement by key players such as church pastors, dedicated church members, and strong leadership by an engaged nurse academic with a commitment to bettering lives in her community. Larger entities such as local farmers and grocers also supported the program, which allowed these vendors to be seen as being interested in the health of their community and generated rewards for them in the form of complimentary advertising for their organizations.

Discussion

Case studies such as this one demonstrate ways in which nurses can become more involved in social justice and advocacy to improve health at a practice level. In order to do so, nurses must focus more attention on tackling the social determinants of heath. Downstream approaches that target individual lifestyle factors (e.g., behavior changes) and provider cultural competence alone, while useful in clinical contexts, have demonstrated very little effect on reducing population inequities because they do not target broader social circumstances as an upstream approach would (Baum & Fisher, 2014; Drevdahl, Canales, & Shannon Dorcy, 2008). An upstream approach recognizes and responds to the roots of health problems, such as improving the social situations and environments that contribute to poorer health outcomes (Braveman, Egerton, & Williams, 2011). Gehlert and colleagues (2008) also address this:

> Although a host of hereditary and individual behavioral factors are linked to health outcomes, we now understand that social circumstances and environmental factors place minority groups at a distinct disadvantage in health and disease. These groups may be exposed to numerous conditions (such as discrimination and unequal treatment in housing, employment, and medical care) experienced less often by more advantaged groups. As such, societal factors that represent upstream determinants should be included in frameworks for determining population health. (p. 340)

Addressing social determinants of health and root causes of health inequities can stem the tide of the increasing health divide between different groups of people. The World Health Organization (2008) has called for primary health care, which includes social justice and advocacy. The nursing profession is well positioned to advance both of these in support of health equity.

Although the AACN promotes curriculum threads of social justice, more scholarship in how to teach social justice at every level of nursing education is needed. For example, by using case studies such as the MTFH in classes, students receive a multidimensional perspective on social justice praxis and can see an upstream approach to public health intervention in action at the local level. In this way, students can envision how social justice and advocacy work in practice.

Social justice is not achieved through one act but must be a continuum of actions at the social, institutional, and policy levels. In addition to understanding concepts of health equity and social justice, the AACN and the ANA call for nurses to advocate for institutional and national policies that address the systemic causes of health inequity. To do this, nurses need to develop a deeper awareness of political processes and policy structures (Carey & Crammond, 2015). In addition to gaining knowledge and skills about advocacy at the institutional and policy levels, nurses also need to realize how institutional and policy change can be influenced in practical and accessible ways.

When engaging in social justice work and advocacy for health equity in any setting, nurses must first acknowledge their role in providing care that recognizes and addresses the social determinants of health. The broader context of a client's life must be explored in each health circumstance in order to design nursing interventions that have the potential for long-term change. Nurses cannot advocate for patients in these broader contexts without developing partnerships that bring about multilevel social change and build health equity capacities (Yanicki et al., 2014).

Just as the World Health Organization calls for nursing leadership in primary health care and the pursuit of health equity, leaders in the field of nursing should enthusiastically voice their support for community engagement and partnership with individual community members, academic organizations and educators, stakeholders, local activists, and policy makers to develop best practices for social justice in primary health care (Yanicki et al., 2014). Health inequities research, the role of primary health care as a strategy for global social justice, and the ANA professional code of ethics no longer allow nurses to see themselves on the sidelines of advocacy and social justice (Thompson, 2014). It is imperative that nurse educators, clinicians, and researchers embrace social justice and advocacy and invoke upstream approaches to address health inequities.

Chapter Activities

1. Explore the different case studies on the Robert Wood Johnson Foundation website: The Role of Primary Care Providers in Changing the Culture of Care in Communities (http://www.rwjf.org/en/culture-of-health/2014/06/the_role_of_primary.html).

   Pick one case study and explore these questions:

   a. How did this case study use the lens of social justice and advocacy in designing their programs?

   b. Multilevel strategies are necessary for promoting social justice. List some of the interventions used in your case study to address health injustices.

2. In your primary health care role, list three ways you can use advocacy to address health inequities in the population you serve.

References

Allender, A. A., Rector, C., & Warner, K. D. (2010). *Community health nursing: Promoting & protecting the public's health* (7th ed.). Philadelphia: Walters, Kluwer, Lippincott, Williams & Wilkins.

American Association of Colleges of Nursing. (1996). *The essentials of master's education for advanced practice nursing.* Retrieved from http://www.aacn .nche.edu/education-resources/essential-series

American Association of Colleges of Nursing. (2006). *The essentials of doctoral education for advanced nursing practice.* Retrieved from http://www.aacn .nche.edu/education-resources/essential-series

American Association of Colleges of Nursing. (2008). *The essentials of baccalaureate education for professional nursing practice.* Retrieved from http://www.aacn .nche.edu/education-resources/essential-series

American Association of Colleges of Nursing. (2011). *The essentials of master's education in nursing.* Retrieved from http://www.aacn.nche.edu/education -resources/essential-series

American Nurses Association. (2015). *Code of ethics for nurses: With interpretive statements.* Maryland: Author.

Anderson, J. M., Rodney, P., Reimer Kirkham, S., Browne, A. J., Khan, K. B., & Lynam, M. J. (2009). Inequities in health and healthcare viewed through the ethical lens of critical social justice: Contextual knowledge for the global priorities ahead. *Advances in Nursing Science, 2009*(4), 282–294.

Baum, F., & Fisher, M. (2014). Why behavioural health promotion endures despite its failure to reduce health inequities. *Sociology of Health and Illness, 36*(2), 213–225.

Bekemeier, B., & Butterfield, P. (2005). Unreconciled inconsistencies: A critical review of the concept of social justice in 3 national nursing documents. *Advances in Nursing Science, 28*(2), 152–162.

Benner, B., Sutphen, Leonard, V., & Day, L. (2010). *Educating nurses: A call for radical transformations.* San Francisco: Jossey-Bass Publishers.

Boutain, D. M. (2004). Social justice in nursing: A review of literature. In M. de Chesnay (Ed.), *Caring for the vulnerable* (pp. 21–29). Sudbury, MA: Jones and Bartlett.

Boutain, D. M., McNees, M., & Moving Together in Faith and Health Collaborative. (2013). Initiating policy, systems, and environmental changes for childhood obesity prevention by engaging six faith-based organizations. *Family and Community Health 36*(3), 248–259.

Braveman, P. (2014). What are health disparities and health equity? We need to be clear. *Public Health Reports, 129*(S2), 5–8.

Braveman, P. A., Kumanyika, S., Fielding, J., Laveist, T., Borrell, L. N., Manderscheid, R., & Troutman, A. (2011). Health disparities and health equity: The issue is justice. *American Journal of Public Health, 101*(Suppl 1), S149–S155.

Braveman, P., Egerton, S., & Williams, D. R. (2011). The social determinants of health: Coming of age. *Annual Review of Public Health, 32*, 381–398.

Buettner-Schmidt, K., & Lobo, M. L. (2012). Social justice: A concept analysis. *Journal of Advanced Nursing, 68*(4), 948–958.

Canales, M. (2000). Othering: Toward an understanding of difference. *Advances in Nursing Science, 22*(4), 16–31.

Carey, G., & Crammond, B. (2015). Action on the social determinants of health: Views from inside the policy process. *Social Science & Medicine, 128*, 134–141.

Chafey, K., Rhea, M., Shannon, A. M., & Spencer, S. (1998). Characterizations of advocacy by practicing nurses. *Journal of Professional Nursing, 14*(1), 43–52.

Chinn, P. L., & Kramer, M. K. (2008). Integrated theory and knowledge development in nursing (7th ed.). St. Louis, MO: Mosby Elsevier.

Day, L. (2010). Health care reform, health, and social justice. *American Journal of Critical Care, 19*(5), 459–461.

Drevdahl, D. J. (2013). Injustice, suffering, difference: How can community health nursing address the suffering of others? *Journal of Community Health Nursing, 30*(1), 49–58.

Drevdahl, D. J., Canales, M. K., & Shannon Dorcy, K. (2008). Of goldfish tanks and moonlight tricks: Can cultural competency ameliorate health disparities? *Advances in Nursing Science, 31*(1), 13–27.

Editorials: The domestic educator and the immigrant. (1913, September). *The Johns Hopkins Nurses Alumnae Magazine, 12*(3), 178–181.

Falk-Rafael, A. (2005). Speaking truth to power: Nursing's legacy and moral imperative. *Advances in Nursing Science, 28*(3), 212–223.

Falk-Rafael, A., & Betker, C. (2012). Witnessing social injustice downstream and advocating for health equity upstream: "The trombone slide" of nursing. *Advances in Nursing Science, 35*(2), 98–112.

Grace, P. J., & Willis, D. G. (2012). Nursing responsibilities and social justice: An analysis in support of disciplinary goals. *Nursing Outlook, 60*(4), 198–207.

Gehlert, S., Sohmer, D., Sacks, T., Mininger, C., McClintock, M., & Olopade, O. (2008). Targeting health disparities: A model linking upstream determinants to downstream interventions. *Health Affairs, 27*(2), 339–349.

Health Resources and Services Administration [HRSA]. (2010). *The registered nurse population: Findings from the 2008 National Sample Survey of Registered Nurses.* Retrieved from http://bhpr.hrsa.gov/healthworkforce/rnsurveys/rnsurveyfinal.pdf

Ingram, M., Sabo, S., Rothers, J., Wennerstrom, A., & de Zapien, J. G. (2008). Community health workers and community advocacy: Addressing health disparities. *Journal of Community Health, 33*(6), 417–424.

Labonte, R. (1994). Health promotion and empowerment: Reflections on professional practice. *Health Education Quarterly, 21*(2), 253–268.

Luther, B., & Hart, S. (2014). What does the Affordable Care Act mean for nursing? *Orthopaedic Nursing, 33*(6), 305–309.

Mohammed, S. A. (2014). Social justice in nursing pedagogy: A postcolonial approach to American Indian health. In P. N. Kagan, M. C. Smith, & P. L. Chinn (Eds.), *Philosophies and practices of emancipatory nursing: Social justice as praxis* (pp. 205–217). New York: Routledge.

Mohammed, S. A., Cooke, C. L., Ezeonwu, M., & Stevens, C. A. (2014). Sowing the seeds of change: Social justice as praxis in undergraduate nursing education. *Journal of Nursing Education, 53*(9), 488–493.

Pauly, B. M., MacKinnon, K., & Varcoe, C. (2009). Revisiting "who gets care?" Health equity as an arena for nursing action. *Advances in Nursing Science, 32*(2), 118–127.

Reimer Kirkham, S., & Anderson, J. M. (2010). The advocate-analyst dialectic in critical and postcolonial feminist research: Reconciling tensions around scientific integrity. *Advances in Nursing Science, 33,* 196–205.

Reimer Kirkham, S., & Browne, A. J. (2006). Toward a critical theoretical interpretation of social justice discourses in nursing. *Advances in Nursing Science, 29*(4), 324–339.

Robert Wood Johnson Foundation. (2014). *Social determinants of health.* Retrieved from http://www.rwjf.org/en/our-topics/topics/social-determinants-of-health.html

Thompson, J. L. (2014). Discourses of social justice: Examining the ethics of democratic professionalism in nursing. *Advances in Nursing Science, 37*(3), E17–E34.

United States Department of Health and Human Services. (2011). *Building healthier communities by investing in prevention.* Retrieved from http://www.hhs.gov .offcampus.lib.washington.edu/healthcare/facts/factsheets/2011/09/prevention02092011.html

United States Department of Health and Human Services. (2014). *Healthy people 2020. Social determinants.* Retrieved from https://www.healthypeople .gov/2020/leading-health-indicators/2020-lhi-topics/Social-Determinants

World Health Organization. (2007, August 16). *The contribution of primary health care to millennium development goals.* Opening address at the International Conference on Health for Development. Buenos Aires, Argentina. Retrieved from http://www.who.int/dg/speeches/2007/20070816_argentina/en/

World Health Organization. (2008) *Primary health care: Now more than ever.* Retrieved from http://www.who.int/whr/2008/en/

Yanicki, S. M., Kushner, K. E., & Reutter, L. (2014). Social inclusion/exclusion as matters of social (in)justice: A call for nursing action [Epub ahead of print]. *Nursing Inquiry.* doi: 10.1111/nin.12076

Zolnierek, C. (2012). Speak to be heard: Effective nurse advocacy. *American Nurse Today, 7*(10). Retrieved from http://www.americannursetoday.com/speak-to -be-heard-effective-nurse-advocacy/

Chapter 5

The Economics of Caring for Populations: A Primary Health Care Perspective

Donna M. Nickitas

Chapter Objectives

By the completion of this chapter, you will be able to:

1. Define an economic and social value framework for nursing practice.
2. Discuss the economics of primary health care.
3. Describe examples of innovative care models developed and implemented by the American Academy of Nurses Edge Runners.

Background

This chapter addresses the economic implications of caring for populations through a nursing social and economic value framework using a primary health care perspective. This perspective addresses the social determinants of health with a focus on underserved and vulnerable populations and espouses that all individuals and communities, but especially vulnerable populations, must have access to affordable health care and opportunities that promote their health and wellness. Improving health care in the United States using this primary health care perspective requires the pursuit of three aims: improving the experience of care, improving the health of populations, and reducing per capita costs of health care (Berwick, Nolan, & Washington, 2008). The Institute for Healthcare Improvement (IHI) developed the Triple Aim as a statement of purpose for fundamentally new health systems that contribute to the overall health of populations while reducing costs (Stiefel & Nolan, 2012, p. 2)

For the purposes of this chapter, the term "population" emerges from the work by Jacobson and Teutsch (2012), who describe the useful distinction of a population as total population or a subpopulation. A total population reflects the residents of a geopolitical area in which a subpopulation may reside. Subpopulations consist of groups defined by income, race/ethnicity, disease burden, or served by a particular health system or workforce such as registered professional nurses or advanced practiced nurses. In either case, it is essential to specify the population so that nurses and other health providers work toward fulfillment of the Triple Aim, which includes partnership with communities and populations with the intent of redesigning primary care of population health toward a care model of improved financial management and macro system integration.

The integration of macro health systems will require nurses to have a care perspective that aligns population health care with better health, better outcomes, and lower costs of care. This macro level integration identifies and includes the Triple Aim outcome measures (Stiefel & Nolan, 2012) of health outcomes, disease burden, and behavioral and physiological factors. These measures are important as they address how care is delivered and how outcomes of care are measured. "Nurses are positioned to be at the forefront of crucial healthcare reform to profoundly affect health outcomes and reduce health disparities" (Mahony & Jones, 2015, p. 283).

With adoption of the Patient Protection and Affordable Care Act (ACA, 2010), there is a resurgence of interest in measures that address the social determinants of health (SDH) and how to improve health status (Mahony & Jones, 2015). In fact, Title IV of the ACA mandates improved disease prevention and public health systems, increased access to preventive services, and provisions for healthier communities, with recognition and attention to the SDH. The World Health Organization (WHO, 2015) defines the social determinants as "the conditions in which people are born, grow, live, work, and age, including the health system. These circumstances are shaped by the distribution of money, power, and resources at global, national, and local levels…"

Addressing the social determinants of health as well as other factors such as poverty, unequal access to health care, lack of education, stigma, and racism provides a greater understanding of how the social determinants affect the health of populations. Nurses must learn how best to understand and recognize the effects of poverty, economic inequities, stress, social exclusions, and job insecurity within populations, especially with those who are medically underserved and most vulnerable (Mahony & Jones, 2015).

When nurses and other health care providers, consumers, and communities are informed and educated about population health, they can transition their focus from federal and state initiatives to local efforts that create conditions for health at their own community level—the level where people work, play, and live. This transition requires a greater understanding about income, education, and where people live as potential predictors of health as well as investing in health care delivery systems that address social determinants of health as a driving force to optimize health, health care quality, and health equity. For example, the Robert Wood Johnson Foundation (RWJF) has made a commitment to advance the nation's health through a movement toward "a culture of health" to address health disparities and health equity specifically within the context of the social determinants of health (Plough, 2014). Developing a culture of health (COH) requires a valuable link between primary health care and population health as well as community services and policies that foster a culture of health. As full partners with physicians and other health professionals in redesigning health care in the United States, nurses play a key role in promoting a culture of health and a steadfast commitment to advancing the nation's health (IOM, 2011).

To improve the health of populations, a framework must be adopted that takes into account the SDH as well as accounting for nursing's economic impact and social values. Using such a framework will achieve the common goals of quality, efficiency, and cost savings in meeting the primary health care needs of underserved and vulnerable populations. For nurses to engage and effectively influence populations, they must be able to assess the effects of SDH and learn how to use this framework to affect the economic and social values of nursing to shape health programs toward population primary health care.

Nursing's Economic and Social Value Framework

Social Value Framework

Nursing's social value can be framed within a primary health care perspective that addresses the social determinants of health and prevents health conditions from developing among underserved or vulnerable populations.

Embedded in these social values are advocacy, cultural sensitivity, social justice, and a population-focused practice framework aligned with the World Health Organization's (WHO, 2008) call to reduce health disparities as well as with the Institute of Medicine's (IOM, 2012) integration of primary health care. In this social value framework, public health is a shared goal of population health improvement and community engagement to define and address population health needs.

Nurses have strong historical roots in advocacy and action that includes determining how to best distribute resources to populations (Lewenson & Nickitas, 2016). Public health nurses have contributed, and continue to contribute strategically in population-based efforts to enhance care. They use data to influence public policy and have a rich heritage of using such data to improve health outcomes (McBride, 1993). This practice dates back to Florence Nightingale, who demonstrated the relationship between data and improvement in care through statistical analysis and graphic representation (Goldwater & Zusy, 1990). Knowing how to use measurable metrics to drive improvements in population health will fundamentally reshape how care is delivered, including evolving toward value-based payments that increase quality at lower costs.

Nursing's Economic Framework

Today, the majority of health care decisions are best understood as economic decisions or at least as having key economic components (Chang, Price, & Pfoutz, 2001). Nursing's economic value and contribution to utilization costs and payer information cannot be underestimated and has real impact on the financial viability of the health care system. As health care costs increase, and efforts to improve the efficiency and effectiveness of the health care system occur, nurses must have a better understanding of health economics. "Economic value of professional nursing refers to a monetary assessment of the services provided by nurses" (Dall, Chen, Seifert, Maddoox, & Hogan, 2009, p. 97). Each nurse must understand his or her economic value and identify and measure that value within the broader context of nursing's value beyond just reduction in health care spending. It is time for every nurse to become a nurse economist (Nickitas, 2011).

In fact, in her book *Notes on Nursing*, Florence Nightingale suggests that nurses have an obligation to understand the financial aspects of patient care (Chang et al., 2001). They must take into account how their human capital (knowledge, expertise, and skills) contributes to ensuring cost-effective, high-quality care (Patterson, 1992). Furthermore, Keepnews (2013) suggests that an improved understanding of nursing's economic value is a tool for explicating and asserting nursing's broad value, both economic and social. This value is essential for "nursing's identity as a discipline focused on care and compassion and key to the professional's social contract "(Keepnews, 2013, p. 2). However, social values alone are not enough; nurses must have the economic acumen of health care finance and understand how the economics of care drive behavior, value, and consumption of health care.

New metrics from electronic health records (EHRs) provide an opportunity to measure nursing care in ways that previously had not been possible. This emerging information across health care settings, from acute care to primary population care in the community, can be used to inform operational and clinical decision-making (Welton & Harper, 2015). Much of nursing care measures, values, and costs remain unknown. For example, in ambulatory or public health in the primary care population model, nursing care costs are captured and subsumed within procedure codes for bundled payment or fee-for-service reimbursement. This means that health insurance and the health care industries seek reimbursement for care when doctors and other health care providers receive a fee for each service (such as an office visit, test, procedure, or other health care service) or by a bundled payment—also known as episode-based payment, episode payment, episode-of-care payment, case rate, evidence-based case rate, global bundled payment, global payment, package pricing, or packaged pricing—which is defined as the reimbursement of health care providers (such as hospitals and physicians) on the basis of expected costs for clinically defined episodes of care (Cromwell, Dayoff, & Thoumaian, 1997; Miller, 2009; Satin & Miles, 2009).

Pappas (2013) challenges nurses to ask: Where do we fit in the care value equation, and how will nurses improve overall population health, achieve better experience, and lower cost? "The variation in nursing resources provided are unknown and there is no alignment among nursing direct-care time and costs, billing for nursing services, and payment for care" (Welton & Harper, 2015, p. 14). It is the profession's collective responsibility and effort to describe what constitutes the components of nursing care value and how best to cost out nursing services wherever nursing care occurs. Costing out nursing services will require that nurses master the fundamentals of health care finance.

Health Care Finance

Health care financing is a challenging topic but not impossible to understand. It is essential that each nurse, regardless of his or her position, understands the economics of care and how the Affordable Care Act will affect health care economics. Health economics is defined as a branch of economics concerned with issues related to effectiveness, value, and behavior in the production and consumption of health and health care (Altarum Institute, n.d.). It is important to note that health care production includes both the component of distribution, in this case across populations, as well as resources allocated within the health economy. Thus, within the production process is health care spending. Health spending is a combination of a product of the *price* of health care services and the *utilization* of those services. Price and utilization are the key drivers of overall health care spending in the United States.

The United States spent $2.9 trillion on health care in 2013, or about $9,255 per person, according to a new detailed accounting of the nation's health care dollars. "The share of gross domestic product devoted to health care spending has remained at 17.4 percent since 2009. Health care spending decelerated 0.5 percentage point in 2013, compared to 2012, as a result of slower growth in private health insurance and Medicare spending. Slower growth in spending for hospital care, investments in medical structures and equipment, and spending for physician and clinical care also contributed to the low overall increase" (Hartman, Martin, Lassman, Catlin, & National Health Expenditure Accounts Team, 2015, p. 1150).

The Centers for Medicare and Medicaid Services (CMS) estimate that American health spending will reach nearly $5 trillion, or 20% of GDP, by 2021 (Ginsburg et al., 2012). An analysis of Medicare spending from 2000 to 2011 found that in 2011 per capita spending increased with age, from $7,566 for beneficiaries age 70, to $16,145 at age 96, and then declined for even older beneficiaries (Neuman, Cubanski, & Damico, 2015).

Nursing Care and Health Care Spending

Health care spending is being influenced by the delivery reforms as a result of the Affordable Care Act, which is altering care patterns and spending for populations with significant health needs. One of the provisions of the ACA is to develop a national quality improvement strategy that will improve delivery of services and population health outcomes. Nurses are leading with care models and strategies that are improving care management for high-need vulnerable populations by better care management and care coordination, which reduce preventable hospitalizations. Through evidence-based care, improved analytics, and metrics to measure outcome, nurses are controlling cost of care as well as meeting the challenges of economic accountability. The real challenge now is how best to engage, empower, and entrust that each nurse becomes accountable to the economic liabilities of poor care, readmission penalties, and preventable errors such that investment toward quality population primary health care are fully realized and rewarded. Nurses must appreciate how the costs of quality primary health care generate potential savings and sustain population health. The economics of care are built upon an understanding and acceptance that every care encounter is a return on investment in an individual, family, or population's health and well-being.

Nurses have a stake in transforming America's fragmented, expensive, and often inaccessible health care system. The American Academy of Nursing's (n.d.) Raise the Voice campaign has promoted and published primary health care models generated by nurses on their website. These care models have the potential to save the health care system money, reduce adverse events, improve patient and population outcomes, and promote health. It is time for a new health care delivery system that focuses on population health and wellness and uses nursing's economic and social value system to shift care away from hospitals and into communities, creating systems where nursing units of service, interventions, procedures, surveillance, and assessments are valued and population health outcomes are improved and adverse events reduced.

In fact, nurses have developed innovative models of care that are adding value to health care by improving financial savings as well as improving quality, safety, and better outcomes for patients, families, and populations in their home communities. Some of these innovative models of care are known as *Edge Runners*, named by the American Academy of Nurses (n.d.) for nurses who were known to develop and implement practice models to promote and manage illness across diverse and underserved populations. Edge Runners have developed care models and interventions that demonstrate significant clinical and financial outcomes. These nurse-led care models are team-based approaches that ensure better health through care coordination. Nurse-led care models improve efficiency through care coordination. The Agency for Healthcare Research and Quality (AHRQ, 2014) defines care coordination as care that deliberately organizes patient care activities and shares information among all the participants concerned with a patient's care to achieve safer and more effective care.

An essential aspect of Edge Runner care models is care coordination, an essential part of professional nursing practice and one of the standards of practice for nurses. It is aimed at providing and managing care needs along the continuum of care and across different settings. Good care coordination supports population primary health care that aligns with the Affordable Care Act by bundling acute and postacute payments and incentivizing value-based care. Incentives for innovation and improvement for care coordination must be recognized. Paying for quality performance is an essential component of the nursing economic framework. To the extent that nurses demonstrate and link quality outcomes to improved care coordination, eliminate error and complications, and eliminate waste, nursing's social value is fully realized. Continued efforts must be made to identify and define both the economic and social value of nursing. Every nurse must recognize the economic and social value his or her clinical practice and stay abreast of health care finance, including how knowledge and practice adds value and provides cost savings.

When nurses are accountable both clinically and economically, they shape their nursing practice models toward improvement and away from financial catastrophe. Clinical care is accountable when population preferences are respectful and responsive to the needs of the populations served. The imperative for nurses is to link population preferences and needs to lower costs.

Edge Runner Models of Care

The key to lowering health care costs is to provide models of care that improve efficiency and effectiveness in how services are delivered. For care to be truly valued and determined to have economic value within the health care system, it must promote the value of the registered nurse in caring for vulnerable populations and using care coordination. The Nurse-Family Partnership (NFP) and the Transitional Model of Care (TMC) have demonstrated significant economic, social, and clinical value. In both cases, these models have focused on the specialized needs of a population. The NFP is a community-based program, and nurses work with first-time low-income mothers or vulnerable mothers from pregnancy until the child is 2 years old. The NFP programs have spread to 800 cities and towns, reaching more than 115,000 mothers and children (Tavernise, 2015). Nurses make home visits, helping mothers gain the confidence to care for themselves and their child. The NFP has been estimated to save $9,118 per child and as much as $26,298 as a return to society, for a net return savings of $17,180 (Karoly, Kilburn, & Cannon, 2005).

The TMC was developed and implemented by Mary Naylor, PhD, RN, FAAN, of the University of Pennsylvania School of Nursing. It has used advanced practice registered nurses (APRNs) to facilitate transitions across care settings (from in-patient to out-patient/home) successfully to reduce hospital readmissions and lower cost. The TMC is a well-designed approach that delivers care to the right people at the right time to improve outcomes for everyone: patients, providers, and payers. The TMC initially focused on comprehensive in-hospital planning and home follow-up for the population of chronically ill, high-risk older adults who have been hospitalized—as well as their family caregivers. It now has expanded to prevent hospitalization of community-dwelling older adults.

It is important for nurses to appreciate and recognize how nurse-led models of care make a difference. Nurse-led models of care focus on wellness, primary health care, and prevention rather than on traditional acute or episodic care. As health care delivery shifts from fee-for-service models of care to value-based models, nurses are well positioned to use clinical and administrative data to measure nursing care, the quality of that care, and patient satisfaction with that care (Nickitas, 2014). The NFP has effectively harnessed the value of clinical and financial data to illustrate how nurses are tackling important health problems and rigorously evaluating them. This care model demonstrates that nurses are using their economic and social value to drive change toward care, quality outcomes, and equity, and it has caught the attention of President Obama, who has funded the program on a national scale since 2010. Such visiting programs have been paid for through the Affordable Care Act (Tavernise, 2015). These outcomes are addressing the persistently high rates of infant mortality while improving quality of life for mothers and infants, as well as increasing productivity and satisfaction for nurses.

Population Primary Health Care and the Affordable Care Act

The Affordable Care Act (ACA) has provided unique opportunities for nurses to create models of care that improve the public's health, including provisions that improve access to care and quality care, while controlling costs. There are many new initiatives to expand access to health care coverage and services for tens of millions of Americans. In fact, since the open enrollment period in 2013 for federal and state health insurance exchanges as a provision of the ACA, approximately 16 million Americans gained coverage, and that number is expected to grow to an estimated 30 to 34 million in the next few years (Clipper, 2015).

To promote a population primary care health model, nurses have a moral and ethical obligation to understand the key social determinants of health care and to seek effective ways to distribute resources to populations to meet their primary health care needs. This means addressing care gaps and avoiding service duplication. Population health outcomes have been identified in the ACA for actual demonstration projects that can be adapted as models of care and resonate with a primary health care perspective.

With the insurance expansion and increased access to population primary health care demand, the nursing workforce is well positioned to meet this demand through demonstration projects and primary care initiatives. Advanced practice registered nurses (nurse practitioners, certified nurse-midwives, certified registered nurse anesthetists, and clinical nurse specialists) provide safe, high-quality, effective care. By utilizing APRNs to the full extent of their education and training, nurses can augment the delivery system and transform health care so it is accessible to all, promoting wellness, managing chronic diseases, and improving health outcomes. Increasing access and expanding population primary health care is possible with a nursing workforce that is prepared and oriented toward a value-based health care payment system. A value-based system replaces the traditional fee-for-service system with metrics focused on better care and better outcomes at lower costs.

Advanced practice registered nurses, specifically primary care nurse practitioners (NPs), have the capacity to care for underserved and vulnerable populations. It is important to note that although APRNs contribute high-quality services across the continuum of care, they are not reimbursed or paid at the same service level as physicians. Not all NPs have a national provider identifier (NPI) for billing purposes. The NPI, or the practice of incident of billing, makes it possible to distinguish the services provided by the NP from those provided by the MD. "Under the incident of billing, physicians bill Medicare using their own NPI services that were actually provided by the NP" (Buerhaus, DesRoches, Dittus, & Donelan, 2015, p. 151). For example, nurse practitioners and clinical nurse specialists (CNs) are paid by Medicare at 85% of the amount that would be paid to physicians for the same level of services.

The payment or reimbursement model is a barrier to APRN practice. It affects both the economic and social value framework of nursing. The Centers for Medicare and Medicaid Services cannot differentiate the incident of billing to NPs, when billed under the MD provider, and are unable to account for the quality and costs of the APRN. APRN services are assigned a lower value than physician services. This barrier raises a problem for Americans who are seeking to enroll in federal and state insurance exchanges as a result of the ACA and gain access to care by APRNs. To change reimbursement policy for APRNs and remove outdated policies by insurance companies will require all professional nurses to be informed and educated about how third-party payers arrange direct reimbursement to APRNs who are practicing within their scope of practice under state law. APRNS deserve to be reimbursed at 100% of the Physician Fee Schedule, especially as expanded access from the ACA brings many more underserved and vulnerable populations to the health care market.

The Affordable Care Act focuses on preventive health care with much attention to supporting primary health care. By law, all citizens must have a primary care provider by 2014 (ACA, 2010). By promoting primary care and a population primary health care model, nurses are at the front line of health care reform. Through population-focused cared, health disparities and social determinants of health can be fully addressed. Underserved and vulnerable populations can become actively engaged in their own care, which in turn increases the effectiveness of the population primary health care model.

Conclusion

From unmet primary health care needs to the high-need, high-cost of preventable hospitalizations, the economic and human suffering of poor access to care to underserved and vulnerable populations where they live, work, and play has enormous financial costs. Clear and abundant evidence shows that primary health care improves overall health and well-being. Targeted application of preventive services, based on unique patient history and evidence-based practice, may be a more cost-effective way to promote health and prevent disease (Goetzel, 2009).

Today nurses are expected to deliver care across different settings, increase patient and provider satisfaction, reduce hospitalizations, and enhance cost savings (Naylor, et al., 2013). To accomplish this, nurses must be ready to step up to the challenge to identify and quantify their economic and social value. There are increasing opportunities to practice at the top of their professional license (IOM, 2011) and to affect the culture of health as never before. The sure way to accomplish this is for nurses to continue to develop and implement models of care that include population primary health care. These models are unique to nursing and focus on improved patient outcomes at lower cost. The economics of care for populations supported and embedded in the ACA are for prevention and wellness as well as for improving quality and how health system performance is measured and evaluated. Nurse-led models of care and nurses practicing population primary health care are well positioned to demonstrate quality measures that improve delivery of services, outcomes, and population health. The long-term objective of population health is to leverage nursing practice to places where people live, work, and play to improve quality and safety and to reduce the costs of health care.

Chapter Activities

1. Discuss the impact the ACA has had on nursing practice and be ready to present (or "pitch") this to your colleagues.
2. Reflect on your own understanding of how economics affects primary health care.

References

Affordable Care Act, read the law. (2010). Retrieved from http://www.hhs.gov/healthcare/rights/law/index.html

Agency for Healthcare Research and Quality. (n.d.). *Care coordination, quality improvement.* Retrieved from http://www.ahrq.gov/research/findings/evidence-based-reports/caregaptp.html

Altarum Institute. (n.d.). *Health economics.* Retrieved from http://altarum.org/areas-of-expertise/health-economics

American Academy of Nursing. (n.d.). *Edge runner.* Retrieved from http://www.aannet.org/edgerunners

Berwick, D. M., Nolan, T. W., & Washington, J. (2008). The triple aim: Care, health, and cost. *Health Affairs, 27,* 759–769. doi:10.1377/hlthaff.27.3.759

Buerhaus, P. I., DesRoches, C. M., Dittus, R., & Donelan, K. (2015). Practice characteristics of primary nurse practitioners and physicians. *Nursing Outlook, 63*(2), 144–143.

Chang, C. F., Price, S. A., & Pfoutz, S. K. (2001). *Economics and nursing: Critical professional issues.* Philadelphia: F. A. Davis Company.

Clipper, B. (2015, September 23). What the ACA means for nursing for a year after open enrollment. *The American Nurse.* Retrieved from http://www.theamericannurse.org/index.php/2015/01/05/what-the-aca-means-for-nursing-a-year-after-open-enrollment/

Cromwell J., Dayhoff, D. A., & Thoumaian, A. H. (1997). Cost savings and physician responses to global bundled payments for Medicare heart bypass surgery. *Health Care Finance Review, 19*(1), 41–57.

Dall, T. M. Chen, Y. J., Seifert, R. F., Maddox, P. J., & Hogan, P. F. (2009). The economic value of professional nursing. *Medical Care, 47*(1), 97–104.

Ginsburg, P., Hughes, M., Adler, L., Burke, S., Hoagland, G. W., Jennings, C., & Lieberman, S. (2012). *What is driving U.S. health care spending. America's unsustainable health care cost growth.* Retrieved from http://www.rwjf.org/en/library/research/2012/09/what-is-driving-u-s--health-care-spending.html

Goetzel, R. Z. (2009). Do prevention or treatment services save money? The wrong debate. *Health Affairs, 28*(1), 37–41.

Goldwater, M., & Zusy, M. (1990). *Prescription for nurses effective political action.* St. Louis: Mosby-Year Book.

Hartman, M., Martin, A. B., Lassman, D., Catlin, A., & National Health Expenditure Accounts Team. (2015). The overall economy. *Health Affairs, 34,* 1150–1160.

Institute of Medicine. (2011). *The future of nursing.* Washington, DC: National Academies Press.

Institute of Medicine. (2012). *Primary care and public health: Exploring integration to improve population health.* Washington, DC: National Academies of Practice Press.

Jacobson, D. M., & Teutsch, S. (2012). An environmental scan of integrated approaches for defining and measuring total population health by the clinical care system, the government public health system, and stakeholder organizations. Retrieved from http://www.improvingpopulationhealth.org/PopHealthPhaseIICommissionedPaper.pdf

Karoly, L. A., Kilburn, M. R., & Cannon, J. S. (2005). *Early childhood interventions: Proven results, future promise.* Santa Monica, CA: Rand Corporation.

Keepnews, D. M. (2013). *Mapping the economic value of nursing.* [A White Paper.] Seattle: Washington State Nurses Association.

Lewenson, S. B., & Nickitas, D. M. (2016). Nursing's history of advocacy and action. In D. M. Nickitas, D. J. Middaugh, & N. Aries (Eds.), *Policy and politics for nurses and other health professionals* (2nd ed., pp. 3–13). Burlington, MA: Jones & Bartlett Learning.

Mahony, D., & Jones, E. J. (2015). Social determinants of health in nursing education, research, and health policy. *Nursing Science Quarterly, 26*(3), 280–284.

McBride, M. (1993). From the president: On being opportunistic. *Nursing Outlook, 41*, 275–276.

Miller, H. D. (2009). From volume to value: Better ways to pay for health care. *Health Affairs, 28*(5), 1418–1428.

Naylor, M. D., Bowles, K. H., McCauley, K. M., Maccoy, M. C., Maislin, G., Pauly, M. V., & Krakauer, R. (2013). High-value transitional care: translation of research into practice. *Journal of Evaluation in Clinical Practice, 19*(5), 727–733. doi:10.1111/j.1365-2753.2011.01659.x

Neuman, P., Cubanski, J., and Damico A. (2015). Medicare per capita spending by age and service: new data highlights oldest beneficiaries. *Health Affairs, 34*(2), 335–339. doi: 10.1377/hlthaff.2014.1371..

Nickitas, D. M. (2014). Clinical analytics for data-driven models of care. *Nursing Economics, 32*(3), 106, 165.

Nickitas, D. M. (2011). Every nurse is a nurse economist. *Nursing Economics, 29*(5), 229, 250.

Pappas, S. H. (2013). Value, a nursing outcome. *Nursing Administration Quarterly, 37*(2), 122–128.

Patterson, C. (1992). The economic value of nursing. *Nursing Economics, 10*, 192–204.

Plough, A. L. (2014). Building a culture of health. *American Journal of Preventive Medicine, 47*(5), S388–S390.

Satin, D. J., & Miles, J. (2009). Performance-based bundled payments: Potential benefits and burdens. *Minnesota Medicine, 92*(10), 33–35.

Stiefel M., & Nolan K. (2012). *A Guide to Measuring the Triple Aim: Population Health, Experience of Care, and Per Capita Cost.* IHI Innovation Series white paper. Cambridge, Massachusetts: Institute for Healthcare Improvement. Retrieved from http://www.ihi.org/resources/pages/ihiwhitepapers/aguidetomeasuringtripleaim.aspx

Tavernise, S. (2015, March 9). Visiting nurses helping moms on the margins. *New York Times*, pp. A1, A10.

Welton, J. M., & Harper, E. M. (2015). Nursing care value-based financial models. *Nursing Economics, 33*(1), 14–19, 25.

World Health Organization. (2008). *Commission on Social Determinants of Health final report.* Geneva, Switzerland: World Health Organization, Commission on Social Determinants of Health.

World Health Organization. (2015). Health topics: Social Determinants of Health. Retrieved from http://www.who.int/topics/social_determinants/en/

Coalitions, Partnerships, and Shared Decision-Making: A Primary Health Care Perspective

Marie Truglio-Londrigan

Chapter Objectives

By the end of this chapter, you will be able to:

1. Examine the potential outcomes of coalitions.

2. Contemplate the shared values essential for coalition formation and sustainability.

3. Discuss the importance of individual, family, community, and population participation in relation to the development of culturally congruent coalition-based interventions for positive health outcomes.

4. Analyze the interrelatedness of coalitions, partnerships, and shared decision-making within a primary health care perspective.

In March of 1915 Edna L. Foley, RN, wrote about a visit to Mansfield House in England where meals were served to children under the Provision of Meals Act of 1906. Three meals were served daily to undernourished school-aged children. Much of the work carried out at the Mansfield House, including the meals served, was documented. These reports described additional efforts carried out by other providers of care including medical inspectors, school nurses, an oculist, and a dentist and gives additional insight about the school clinic of the time (Foley, 1915). This article provides a glimpse into the work carried out by different care providers during the early 20th century in an attempt to meet the health care needs of children. Although this work was not a formal partnership or coalition as we understand it today, it does show that those who provided care understood that the most vulnerable required care from multiple providers. These early providers of care understood the need to work together to meet the complex and diverse needs of those most vulnerable.

Today we have expanded our understanding of the need to connect, partner, and collaborate with other care providers, thereby establishing collective action through the development of what we now understand to be coalitions. This chapter provides a forum in which (a) coalitions are defined; (b) the structure and processes of coalitions are explained through the presentation of the Community Coalition Action Theory (CCAT); (c) examples of coalitions are presented; (d) outcomes of coalition initiatives are shared; (e) facilitators of coalition development, implementation, and sustainability are presented; and (f) the perspective of primary health care and the role of coalitions, partnerships, and shared decision-making within this perspective is examined.[1]

Coalitions

Butterfoss (2007) notes that partnerships and coalitions may not have existed in early American culture, but the idea of people coming together, connecting, and collectively sharing resources via community organizations for positive change has always been in existence. Butterfoss further states that the more formal partnership development leading to contemporary coalition formation that builds community competency began to take shape in the 1990s. This community competency takes place as the people in the communities themselves partake in the work of the coalition, known as citizen participation, thereby enhancing community development, community capacity, and empowerment of the people and the community within which the people live (Florin, Mitchell, Stevenson, & Klein, 2000).

---

[1]Portions of this chapter have been taken from Truglio-Londrigan, M., & Barnes, C. (2015). Working together: Shared decision-making. In S. B. Lewenson & M. Truglio-Londrigan (Eds.), *Decision-making in nursing: Thoughtful approaches for leadership* (pp. 141–156). Burlington, MA: Jones & Bartlett Learning.

Definitions

The definitions of coalitions are varied and many illustrate the evolution of the term. Coalitions have traditionally been defined as individuals from varying groups, organizations, and constituencies who come together to form a partnership and who agree to work together to achieve a common goal (Feighery & Rogers, 1990). Sullivan (1998) concurs with this definition and adds that working together to meet a common goal is essential, for without the partnership each individual organization may not be able to achieve its individual goal (Truglio-Londrigan & Barnes, 2015). Berkowitz and Wolff (2000) extend this definition and state that a coalition is "a group involving multiple sectors of the community, coming together to address community needs and solving community problems" (p. 2). Finally, Cohen, Baer, and Satterwhite (2002) identify the coalition as "a union of people and organizations working to influence outcomes on a specific problem" (p. 1). The significance of this definition rests with use of the word "people," which broadens the notion of coalitions by providing a forum for individual community members to be active participants in the coalition. Obtaining local community people's views as coalition members serves to enhance the coalition's abilities to identify community problems, and to more specifically target resources within the community and enhance the people's own "self-confidence, skills and knowledge needed to take advantage of opportunities as they arise" (Ansari & Phillips, 2001, p. 352). Contemplating these definitions highlights several themes. These themes include partnerships, collaboration, and community need. That is, the need for partnerships among individuals, groups, organizations, and communities that are developed and through which people collaborate and respond to a particular identified community need.

Types of Coalitions

Coalitions are varied and operationally different depending on the reason for the coalition, the issue the coalition is responding to, the goal, membership, structure of the coalition, processes of the coalition, and the type of outcomes the coalition membership wishes to achieve. Many types of coalitions are noted in the literature (Truglio-Londrigan & Barnes, 2015). Coalitions may be temporary or more permanent. For example, Feighery and Rogers (1990) identified three types of coalitions. The grassroots coalition is the first of the three types, and it is developed by people who voluntarily organize to address an issue. Second is the professional coalition, which is developed and implemented by professionals. In the professional coalition, a lead organization sets the stage, begins the process, offers resources, and assists in brokering the membership. Third is the community-based coalition, which is developed by professionals as well as community leaders and includes community members to address community-based issues. In this coalition, membership is diverse and may include local organizations such as schools, houses of worship, local nonprofit and for-profit organizations, and recreational organizations. Butterfoss (2007) adds state and regional or national coalitions to this list of types of coalitions. Of particular interest for this text on primary health care is the community-based coalition (Truglio-Londrigan & Barnes, 2015).

Community-Based Coalitions

The community-based coalition provides a way to bring about change and address community-based issues with community members as active participants (Truglio-Londrigan & Barnes, 2015). What makes the community-based coalition different is the active engagement of people from the community who share in all decisions at all stages. Ansari and Phillips (2001) describe the "mutual creation" of the organization and the activities of the organization as being important for a "sense of ownership" (p. 353). In many respects these community-based coalitions are a means for the people in the community to become "agents of social change" and to advance their own agenda (Nelson, Prilleltensky, & MacGillivary, 2001, p. 651).

A key component of a coalition's success is recognizing that community members are experts in understanding the experience of "living in their community" and can offer valuable insight. Actions by people from the community serve to enhance community competency. For example, a professional organization may identify an issue in a community affecting a particular population using data derived from large databases. To address this issue, the professional organization may begin the process of developing a community-based coalition by sharing both their concerns and the data they retrieved and analyzed. People from the community may agree with the professional organization in theory, but they may disagree with using the data from the large databases alone as evidence. The people from the community, who have the experience of living in the community, may have other information or evidence that illustrates another priority problem that needs to be addressed first.

The decision on what issue needs to be worked on is a joint venture, and the final decision made is a shared decision between and among all involved as a result of a negotiation process that involves education and consideration of best practice evidence (Truglio-Londrigan, 2013; Truglio-Londrigan, in press a, in press b; Truglio-Londrigan & Barnes, 2015). Furthermore, through their active and engaged membership in the coalition, community members may also strengthen the work of the coalition in the development of successful intervention strategies to address the community issue. For example, the general membership of the coalition may wish to use a best practice intervention strategy derived from a search of the literature. The coalition members who live in the community and who represent the diverse nature of the community may see inherent problems with implementation of the best practice strategy because the strategy is not culturally sensitive, appropriate, or culturally congruent with their community or the population of interest. In this scenario, the process of negotiation is of equal importance. This type of participation serves as a check to all of the coalition members to stop, listen, and rethink their strategy. In some cases, the coalition may need to take the time to develop a participatory action research project with community members in an attempt to develop best practice that is culturally significant and meaningful for their community and the specific population of interest (Soleimanpour, Brindis, Geierstanger, Kandawalla, & Kurlaender, 2008; Vaughn et al., 2013).

In community-based coalitions, the people in the community are not just interviewed or "tapped into" for information; they are active, engaged, participatory members who share in the decisions of the coalition. They are held responsible and accountable to the other members of the coalition and, most important, to the members within the community whom they represent. The case study that follows illustrates a tertiary care organization that led in the development of a community coalition. This case is an example of the "complex, multi-layered problems that require sophisticated solutions at the community level" and how "coalitions by themselves are not a prevention strategy, but a means whereby a community can organize, plan, and deliver multi-level and multi-faceted prevention programs, policies, and practices" (Center for Prevention Research and Development, 2006, p. 3). This example demonstrates the important place of coalitions within a primary health care perspective (Truglio-Londrigan & Barnes, 2015).

Case Study: Developing a Community Coalition

Yvette Melendez, Vice President, Government and Community Alliances; and Donna Avanecean, Hartford Hospital

Hartford Hospital is an 867-bed tertiary care center and is the largest teaching and referral center in the New England region. It is the flagship hospital of the Hartford Healthcare System, a large and diversified system. Hartford Hospital's vision is to be nationally respected for excellence in patient care and most trusted for personalized coordinated care. Its mission is to improve the health and healing of the people and communities it serves.

Hartford Hospital is located in the city of Hartford with a diverse population of approximately 127,000 of which 42% are Latino, 38% Black, and 31% White. Like many urban centers, economic disparity is significant when compared to the rest of the state. The median income in Hartford is approximately $29,600 as compared to the overall state median of $70,000. The city's poverty rate is 32% compared to a state average of 9%.

Poverty and high unemployment have resulted in health disparities and poor access to health services, and many residents are either uninsured or underinsured. Hartford Hospital is the second largest provider of Medicaid services in the state. These disparities have resulted in a diabetes prevalence rate of 7.6%, obesity rate of 33.9%, and an asthma rate in children of 41%. Over 12% of the residents have poor mental health; the leading cause of death in the city is related to heart disease.

Hartford Hospital has a long history of serving the city and its residents through a variety of community health initiatives. A community health needs assessment identified several opportunities to improve the health status of its residents. African American men were particularly identified as an "at-risk group" for poor health. A collaborative program between Hartford Hospital and the Omega Foundation of Hartford was developed. Originally known as the Black Men's Project, this initiative aimed to empower African American men in the community in caring for themselves and their families by providing educational opportunities and health screening at church halls as well as at local barbershops. A diverse hospital team including a board member, community health nurse, nutritionist, cancer outreach workers, and other health professions, as well as church leaders and barbershop owners, became regulars in one of the most disadvantaged communities in the city. The initiative has provided over 3,000 screenings in approximately 18 months and over 100 men have been referred to primary care providers. A particular case that embodies the impact of this program is the story of JD, a 34-year-old security guard at a local school. JD entered the barbershop one Saturday when the Take Charge program was there. He was at least 80 lbs overweight and was suffering from chronic fatigue. When one of the volunteers took his blood pressure, it was 160/90; JD was scared enough that he committed to change his diet and way of life. With the help of the community nurse, who navigated JD through his doctor's visits and nutrition counseling, and became his health coach, JD has lost over 50 lbs and his current blood pressure is 136/80. He now has a very different diet and has recruited others to the events. He is our best spokesman for the program and for the message to men about assuming responsibility for their own health, with no excuses, no matter how disadvantaged they might feel.

Hartford Hospital continues to value the relationships it has established within the community it serves. In addition to the Black Men's Health Project, Hartford Hospital has developed partnerships in areas such as workforce development, economic development, wellness and health care services, and special events support. At the present time, Hartford Hospital has several special projects including the Southside Institutions Neighborhood Association, Breastfeeding Heritage and Pride Peer Counseling Program, and the Center for Eliminating Health Disparities Among Latinos, to name a few.[*]

Community Coalition Action Theory (CCAT)

The CCAT provides a framework for individuals and organizations who may be interested in developing a community-based coalition to address

---

[*]Reprinted by permission from Yvette Melendez, BA, MS, Vice President, Government and Community Alliances, and Donna Avanecean, RN, FNP-C, CNRN, APRN, Hartford Hospital.

community or population-based issues. From the brief review of the literature pertaining to coalitions and the partnerships inherent within these coalitions, it is evident that the structure and processes of the coalition's organizational framework are indeed complex. To facilitate a greater understanding, Butterfoss and Kegler (2009) and Butterfoss (2007) developed the Community Coalition Action Theory (Truglio-Londrigan & Barnes, 2015). This model, including the structure and process as well as outcomes, are described below.

Structure and Process

Upon initial consideration of this model stages are noted. The stages (formation, maintenance, and institutionalization) are considered the first of fourteen constructs. These stages are cyclical in nature, not linear (Butterfoss, 2007; Butterfoss & Kegler, 2009) and represent the life cycle of a coalition. In the formation stage the lead organization begins the process of identifying the initial community organizations and individuals who will initiate the early work of the coalition. The maintenance stage involves assessments to identify community issues as well as interventions and plans to address issues. The maintenance stage also involves processes that maintain the progress of the intervention strategies and all activities that sustain the coalition work such as education programs. The final institutionalization stage takes place as the evaluation demonstrates achievement of the goals. Butterfoss (2007) asserts that successful strategies may result in changes in knowledge, beliefs, attitudes, and behavior as well as changes in systems, policy, and law.

The CCAT illustrates thirteen additional constructs: community context, lead agency/convener group, coalition membership, operation and processes, leadership and staffing, structures, pooled member and external resources, member engagement, assessment and planning, implementation of strategies, community change outcomes, health/social outcomes, and community capacity (Butterfoss, 2007; Butterfoss & Kegler, 2009). To delve into each of these constructs is beyond the scope of this chapter, but a brief summary follows (Truglio-Londrigan & Barnes, 2015).

First is the need to understand the community contextual factors. For example, knowing the history of a community, understanding how political officials have traditionally operated and voted on past issues, or having an awareness of the relationships between and among defined groups and populations within a community is important. The remaining constructs further define what the coalition is and how the coalition is operationalized. For example, the lead organization, such as a Department of Health, may act as a convener or a broker for the other organizations. The lead organization may host an initial meeting and provide initial support. The initial core group of the community coalition ultimately expands to include a larger more diverse representation of the community, formal and other informal community groups, public and private organizations, and key individuals in the community who may have an interest in the work of the coalition. These community groups, organizations, and individuals may share similar ideas, values, and beliefs pertaining to the identified issue or population and may have a desire to work with the lead organization (Butterfoss, 2007; Butterfoss & Kegler, 2009; Truglio-Londrigan & Barnes, 2015).

The operations and processes of the coalition are soon formalized, including (a) developing vision and mission statements, (b) identifying the process for shared decision-making, (c) instituting communication processes, and (d) discussing conflict management and negotiation processes. Consideration must be given to leadership and staffing and the roles of each. Formalizing the structure of the coalition, including bylaws, policies, and procedures, is important (Butterfoss, 2007; Butterfoss & Kegler, 2009; Center for Prevention Research and Development, 2006; Foster-Fishman, Berkowitz, Lounsbury, Jacobson, & Allen, 2001; Truglio-Londrigan & Barnes, 2015). In addition, consideration of how to build a structure that is neither hierarchical nor autocratic in nature is necessary. A flat structure, in which there is shared dialogue between all members (Truglio-Londrigan & Barnes, 2015), facilitates shared decision-making that ultimately leads to member engagement and empowerment (Hain & Sandy, 2013). As the members of the coalition work together and pool their resources, they create more detailed community and population-based assessments by researching, planning, implementing, and evaluating best practice strategies (Butterfoss, 2007; Butterfoss & Kegler, 2009; Center for Prevention Research and Development, 2006; Foster-Fishman et al., 2001; Truglio-Londrigan & Barnes, 2015). The totality of the diverse assessments carried out by the coalition members will serve to introduce the coalition to other community individuals and organizations who may volunteer or be invited to participate in the work of the coalition (Center for Prevention Research and Development, 2006). Additional external resources may also be identified via these diverse community assessments. Throughout this process, attention is given to communication, collaboration, team work, problem solving, conflict resolution, negotiation, and goal setting, all of which are facilitated via the shared decision-making process, which is supported by trust that grows with time (Butterfoss, 2007; Butterfoss & Kegler, 2009; Center for Prevention Research and Development, 2006; Truglio-Londrigan & Barnes, 2015).

Outcome

As the coalition implements strategies, evaluation determines whether goals have been achieved and whether there have been additional positive outcomes. Formative evaluation takes place throughout the entire implementation process, and summative evaluation is completed at the end of the implementation process (Cohen et al., 2002). Reflection may be formative and summative, as it takes place throughout the coalition initiative and post initiative. Ultimately this reflective process serves to inform the coalition members and is evaluative in nature.

Self-reflection is a multistage process that includes an awareness of an uncomfortable feeling or thought, a critical analysis of the situation including questioning, and the development of a new perspective (Atkins & Murphy, 1993). Schön (2006) introduced the concepts of reflection-in-action and reflection-on-action for reflective practice, and coalition work certainly is a practice that may benefit from individual member and group reflections. Reflection-in-action promotes the belief that members may "think about what we are doing" (Schön, 2006, p. 54) while doing it. As members are individually and collectively thinking about what they are doing, they also are "in the process, evolving their way of doing it" (p. 56). In many respects this reflection-in-action exemplifies formative evaluation.

Reflection-on-action takes place after the interaction, as members "think back on a project they have undertaken, a situation they have lived through, and they explore the understandings they have brought to their handling of the case" (Schön, 2006, p. 61). Coalition members may reflect on their knowledge, behaviors, actions, attitudes, and responses to other members along with looking at how other members are behaving, acting, and responding in relation to them. Self-reflective questioning facilitates members' ability to adjust how they see the work of the coalition and helps them gain greater clarity (Truglio-Londrigan, in press b). This is especially valuable in moments of conflict during shared decision-making.

Evaluation is important in determining whether or not the strategies implemented by the coalition have resulted in the attainment of the established goals and serve to identify additional outcomes. Butterfoss (2007) sees evaluation as "an ongoing process that can help coalition decision makers to better understand their organization and their projects, and how they impact participants, partner agencies, and the community" (p. 436). During the evaluation process many questions are asked (Cohen et al., 2002). If the goal has not been met, has there been progress toward the goal? If the goal has not been met, or if there was only minimal progress, what were the barriers to achievement of the goal? Were there problems in the assessment phase? Were the community member partners of the coalition listened to? Were there problems in communication? Were there enough resources such as financial or educational? If the strategy was an education initiative that was to be delivered to a particular population, was an educational needs assessment conducted first? For example, were the education needs of the population considered in terms of literacy? Can these barriers be addressed? Were there facilitators, and can these facilitators serve to strengthen the work of the coalition? Some additional evaluative questions are included here:

- How satisfied is the population with the intervention strategy that was applied? Did they see the intervention as useful and meaningful? Were they able to gain access to the intervention? If not why not?
- How satisfied are the members of the coalition? Do the members believe that their work was meaningful? Do the members believe that the strategy they developed and implemented was appropriate,

accessible, and acceptable to the population? Do the community members feel that their participation and input was listened to, heard, supported, and appreciated?

- Do the members of the coalition believe their work is representative of the established vision and mission?

- Do the members "see" other successes from their work (Feighery & Rogers, 1990)? For example, in community-based coalitions that include people from the community, there should be a corresponding increase in the community's capacity. Did an individual from the community, who is a coalition member, gain increase knowledge and skills as a result of her or his participation? Did an individual from the community, who is a coalition member, mentor other coalition members the enhance their own capacity for change and growth? Did these individuals then return to their community and mentor others, thus empowering others in the community?

- How has the coalition sustained itself over time (Center for Prevention Research and Development, 2006; Cohen et al., 2002; Foster-Fishman et al., 2001)? Is it the educational programs that they provide for their members? Is it the ability of the coalition to find financial resources? Is it the coalition's ability to search for and recruit new members? Is it the coalition's ability to relate to elected officials?

- Does the community-based coalition evolve with the needs of the community? For example, if a community-based coalition was developed to focus on the needs of the adolescents in the community, is the coalition facile enough to continue to monitor and track what is happening in the community with regard to issues experienced by this population? If, for example, the work of the coalition has traditionally focused on the prevention of alcohol consumption in this population, and there is sudden evidence that another form of drug use is taking place, is the coalition able to effectively and efficiently address this issue and bring it into focus? When evaluating the work of a coalition, their ability to actively respond to a community's needs and address moving targets is critical (Feighery & Rogers, 1990; Gabriel, 2000).

These questions and the answers will guide the coalition in their ongoing work. **Table 6-1** provides examples of coalitions that have been developed and initiated illustrating the population-based issue, coalition development and membership, overarching goal, strategy implementation, and evaluation.

Shared Values and Shared Decision-Making

According to Nelson and colleagues (2001), "Values are guidelines for thinking and acting in ways that benefit others" (p. 652). The values held by the member partners, therefore, facilitate the behavior and actions of the

Table 6-1

Coalition Examples

Source	Description
Pressley, J. C., Barlow, B., Durkin, M., Jacko, S. A., Dominguez, D. R., & Johnson, L. (2005). A national program for injury prevention in children and adolescents: The injury free coalition for kids. *Journal of Urban Health, 82*(3), 389–401.	The Harlem Hospital Injury Prevention Program is an example of a community coalition developed to address injury as a leading cause of death for children. Despite the fact that these injuries are preventable, it has traditionally been neglected. This article presents the development of a community coalition with a vision to reduce injuries and increase the use of safety devices such as booster seats. Initial funding sources included grants from the Robert Wood Johnson Foundation, Centers for Disease Control, local charities, cooperate sponsorship, and philanthropists. Examples of coalition membership include pediatricians, elected public officials, public health professionals, fire and emergency medical personnel, law enforcement, school health and trauma center nurses, parent associations, parents, parks and recreation, and community volunteers. Intervention strategies included educational interventions for safety such as street crossing and fire safety. Education about safety products as well as the distribution of these same products was also incorporated for booster seats and bicycle helmets. Education was directed to specific groups and populations at risk. Overall the incidence of injury among school-aged children declined compared with preintervention rates.
Linowski, S. A., & DiFulvio, G. T. (2012). Mobilizing for change: A case study of a campus and community coalition to reduce high-risk drinking. *Journal of Community Health, 37*(3), 685–693.	This article introduces a campus and community coalition that was developed to address high-risk drinking and the consequences of such drinking. Coalition membership included campus police, town police, town government officials, chamber of commerce, residence life, Greek life, health services, and dean of students, athletics, community relations, and student development. The environmental management strategy implemented by the coalition included activities such as alcohol-free socials, extracurricular activities, public service options, and restriction of marketing and promotion of alcohol on and off campus. Since development and implementation of the environmental strategies, there has been a reduction in student drinking and the consequences of this drinking.

coalition and the shared decisions of the coalition (Truglio-Londrigan & Barnes, 2015). Coalitions have many shared values, some of which are illustrated in **Figure 6-1**.

The overriding vision is the core from which the mission and goals are developed. Together the shared vision, mission, and goals represent the essence of the coalition. It is this shared vision that prompts members of the coalition to act in a collective way, in a partnership, and collaborate without thought of self-interest. Nelson and colleagues (2001) identify this type of partnership as a value-based partnership. In a value-based partnership members all work together to advance "caring, compassion, community, health, self-determination, participation, power sharing, human diversity, and social justice" (p. 651). The value-based partnership illustrates another value of equal importance, which is that the members of a coalition are other centered (Truglio-Londrigan & Barnes, 2015).

The coalition, working together in partnership and collaborating, creates the context for shared decision-making between and among all members of a coalition. The shared decision-making process facilitates "broad

Figure 6-1

Shared Values for Shared Decision-Making
Shared Values of Coalition Members

- Shared Vision
- Shared Mission/Goal
- Collectivism
- Other Centeredness
- Broad Participation
- Inclusiveness
- Respect
- Time
- Self-Reflection
- Share Power With
- Present
- Attentive
- Intention
- Collegiality
- Communication
- Listen
- Value Others

Data from Truglio-Londrigan, M. & Barnes, C. (2015). Working together: Shared decision-making. In S. B. Lewenson & M. Truglio-Londrigan, *Decision-making in nursing: Thoughtful approaches for leadership* (pp. 141–162), Burlington: MA: Jones & Bartlett Learning.

participation in determining the course of the coalition" (Kaye & Wolff, 2002, p. 33). The voices of all members of the coalition must be listened to, heard, and valued, sharing not only in the decision but in the work, including planning, task accomplishments, implementation of strategies, and evaluation of outcomes in a way that exemplifies inclusiveness (Woehrle, 2003). A coalition is nonhierarchical. There is no "power over" in a coalition, only "power with" as members of the coalition exemplify the values of sharing and inclusiveness. Any opposition to this broad participation and inclusiveness inhibits the work of the coalition. Working in coalitions that include individuals from the community is challenging, and hierarchical relationships may develop, which may result in decisions that are not representative of the view of the entire membership of the coalition (Allen, Dyas, & Jones, 2004). This violates the spirit of a coalition (Truglio-Londrigan & Barnes, 2015).

Other values essential for a coalition's work include the need for time to solidify partnerships. Time is essential for relationship development that involves trust and respect. Inclusiveness in the communication exchange between members of the coalition is important and takes time as well. "Exclusion generates [a] 'we-they' dynamic. . . . What is needed is a pluralistic process" (Michaels, 2002, p. 2). Greitemeyer, Schulz-Hardt, Brodbeck, and Frey (2006) note that making decisions in organizations and in life when groups of players participate in the decision-making process requires more time and effort. Members of the coalition must consciously be present, attentive, and listen with intention in every respect. Michaels (2002) speaks to this same issue and notes that through the "practice of listening, intentional speaking, and conscious self-monitoring" (p. 1) consensus will be realized. There is no room for an atmosphere of competition, only collegiality and working together (Truglio-Londrigan & Barnes, 2015). Self-reflection, and the time necessary for self-reflection, enables members of the coalition to become involved in moments of self-checking, asking questions such as these: How do I feel about what is happening? Can I support what is happening? Do I feel listened to? Do I feel that what I have to say is valued? Is the coalition taking on a task that is congruent with the original vision, mission, and goals? Is any one member of the coalition attempting to usurp power? Answers to these questions may give clues to how one feels about the progress and process of the coalition and how one is responding or reacting to others in the coalition at any given moment in time, thus avoiding conflict (Truglio-Londrigan & Barnes, 2015). These self-reflective questions are critical because much of the coalition's work is relational between and among all members of the coalition.

What Does a Coalition Need to Be Successful?

The values and actions required of members shed light on the answer to this question. Coalitions require respect and trust-based relationships, shared decision-making, team work and collaboration, and most certainly the willingness to be accountable and responsible toward the coalition's identified vision and mission statements. Initially, the partnerships within the coalition are held together because of the vision. For example, a community coalition may consist of several health, educational, and social organizations as well as individuals from a particular community who come together to plan and build a skate park for young residents. This skate park may be used by skateboarders and in-liners, which exemplify a particular adolescent population in a given community. Early in the development of the coalition, partnerships within the larger coalition and the relationship between and among all of the members are held together by their vision. In this case, the vision is the need for a safe environment for young residents so they can practice their sport in a safe manner.

The relationship that forms in the development of the coalition reflects a complex network of connections that sets the stage for the development of trust (Goodkind et al., 2011). As the coalition works together and collaborates, over time, trust is reestablished and strengthened (Kang, 1997). Trust facilitates a climate of openness that continually supports the work of the coalition (Porter-O'Grady & Malloch, 2011). This trust is essential because without it the coalition will not be a success (Truglio-Londrigan & Barnes, 2015).

There are many other reasons for a coalition's success. One reason may be a coalition's understanding of the importance of their community members. Community members bring information to the coalition that only they hold. They are the experts on matters of what it is like "living in their community." Their voices bring information that is rich and of great significance. Another reason may be that a coalition's leadership is well versed in understanding how to garner resources, and they have the skills necessary to understand how to negotiate these resources. These resources may include needed funding and technology (Center for Prevention Research and Development, 2006). Furthermore, a coalition's ability to change its vision and mission and how it functions is critical. This has been alluded to earlier with regard to a coalition's ability to meet the challenges of the community's changing needs over time. The ability to engage new membership is also critical for a successful coalition, as individuals leave and migrate out of communities. Coalitions must develop a process to account for this member movement and need to identify processes for searching out and educating new members (Center for Prevention Research and Development, 2006). Finally, it has been noted that shared decision-making is an important process that takes place in coalitions. The process of shared decision-making is complex. The coalition membership may not have the skill-set or the knowledge to engage in the shared decision-making process, so necessary for a coalition's survival. Competencies for shared decision-making are critical aspects in educational programs for coalition members (Truglio-Londrigan, in press b). Foster-Fishman et al. (2001) carried out a qualitative analysis to identify the core competencies and processes necessary for coalition building. These competencies included member capacity, such as the skills and knowledge needed by coalition members that would facilitate their collaboratively working together; relational capacity, such as the development of shared visions and the promotion of power sharing and participatory decision-making; organizational capacity, including leadership, developing effective processes and procedures, including effective communication as well as needed resources; and, finally, addressing programmatic capacity, such as development of goals in alignment with strategies that are based in best practice (Truglio-Londrigan & Barnes, 2015).

Partnerships, Coalitions, and Shared Decision-Making: Ingredients for Primary Health Care

The Primary Health Care Conference in Alma-Ata, Russia, in 1978 introduced the Declaration of Alma-Ata (WHO, 1978). This document asserts the need for all governments to take action to ensure protection and health for all of the people of the world. This document affirms what health is; the inequities of the health of the people of the world between countries and within countries; the importance of economic and social developments in achieving health; the responsibilities of governments to lead; and the responsibilities of the people in the achievement of health through their full and active participation. The declaration continually notes the importance of primary health care (PHC) and the need for the people of the world to be full participants in planning, organizing, and operating services to achieve health. The concepts embedded in the definition of PHC are essential for the work of a coalition.

Concepts in the definition of PHC, such as full participation by all members of a community, are essential ingredients for community-based coalitions. So too are the concepts of self-reliance and self-determination, which are outcomes that illustrate a community's enhanced capacity and a significant positive outcome for a community-based coalition such as the Community Coalition Action Theory. Shared decision-making is exemplified in the mutual partnership with full participation of all member partners, whether those members are from organizations or are individual community members. The partnerships that make up the coalition and the shared decisions made between and among all members of the coalition is the work necessary for the principles of primary health care to be realized. Community-based coalition stories of primary health care in action have the potential to bring about changes in health and health inequities, environment, economic and community development, research driven by community needs, development of acceptable interventions driven by that same community, policy, and social norms creating lasting positive influences for each community.

Conclusion

In today's health care environment, complex problems warrant the development of partnerships and coalitions within the context of PHC. Membership in these coalitions are vast and diverse, and may include private and public organizations, schools, nonprofit and for-profit organizations, recreation facilities, spiritual organizations, health care providers, hospitals and other health care organizations, law enforcement, unions, and people living in the community. The partners within the coalition work together so that the vision, mission, and goals established collectively via shared decision-making become a reality. So important are these coalitions that *Healthy People 2020* offers information on their website pertaining to the development of initiatives using the coalition and consortium frameworks and provides valuable information in their user-friendly tool kits (USDHHS, 2010). Nurses, as leaders, can use this tool kit in the multiple health care settings in which they work to both achieve positive health outcomes and to enhance a community's capacity (Truglio-Londrigan & Barnes, 2015).

Chapter Activity 1

Form a team with your colleagues and carry out the following activities:

1. Identify (a) a population of interest, (b) a community within which this population resides, and (c) a population-based health care issue.

2. Explore the community within which this population resides. You may wish to do a windshield survey or conduct a comprehensive community assessment.

3. Carry out a review of the library databases and gather information about the population-based issue.

4. Explore the determinants of health that place this population at risk for this population-based issue.

5. Carry out a large database search and retrieve incidence, prevalence, morbidity, and mortality data for the population and any important information concerning demographics or determinants of health. It is beneficial to retrieve data for at least 3 decades.

6. Once you have the above information, think creatively and develop a coalition to address the issue.

    ▓ Who will be the members of the coalition, and why have you selected these organizations and individuals to be members (i.e., what is each member's vested interest in participating in the coalition to address the given PHC issue in this population)?

    ▓ Who would be the lead organization? Why?

    ▓ What would be the vision, mission, and goals?

    ▓ What resources would you need?

    ▓ How will you evaluate the work of the coalition?

    ▓ How will you ensure active community participation of the identified population of interest?

    ▓ How will you ensure the sustainability of the coalition?

    ▓ In what ways can you use technology to support the work of the coalition?

Chapter Activity 2

Food Insecurity in the United States Affecting the Most Vulnerable Among Us

By Yaa Boatemaa, Veteran Affairs, Brooklyn, New York

Patient A was admitted to the hospital emergency room. His brother brought him via an ambulance. During the admission assessment, Patient A was not forthcoming with the emergency room doctor who ultimately diagnosed Patient A with altered mental status and established orders to rule out pneumonia and urinary tract infection pending laboratory work, chest X-ray, and EKG. After the emergency room staff completed the assessment, blood draws, and EKG, the patient was sent to the medical/surgical unit.

The admission assessment nurse entered into Patient A's room and sat in a chair next to the bed. This RN introduced herself and began the admission assessment, which included open-ended questions concerning smoking, drinking, and drug intake. The RN also carried out a detailed nutrition assessment because the patient was thin and cachexia. These questions included where the patient lived, who he lived with, where the patient shopped for groceries, the patients financial resources to purchase food, what foods the patient liked to eat, how food is prepared, who prepares food, and whether or not the patient had viable social supports and a social network. Patient A's brother noted that Patient A lived alone and rarely left his apartment to socialize. The brother also stated that on his visit he noted no food in the refrigerator that was eatable and that the remaining food store in the neighborhood that sold fresh fruits, vegetables, and protein sources such as meat and fish closed 3 months prior. After a time Patient A looked at the nurse and stated "there is no place for me to buy food. I cannot travel far to shop in those big supermarkets; I do not drive and it's a problem taking public transportation."

The RN gathered objective data that included a Mini Mental State (MMS). Upon completion of the MMS, no confusion or disorientation was noted and in fact the patient was alert and oriented. The patient was weak, however, and malnourished with poor skin turgor. The remainder of the physical exam was unremarkable, and all tests came back negative for pneumonia and urinary tract infections.

Reflecting on this case, it is easy to see how an older adult may be diagnosed with altered mental status when in fact this may not be the issue plaguing the individual. A misdiagnosis such as this may stay with the older adult interminably while the presiding issue is hidden and continues to cause further problems.

Reflective Questions

- Who is the population?
- What is the population-based issue?
- How would you define food insecurity?
- What information can you locate about food insecurity in the United States?
- How would you develop a coalition in your own community surrounding food insecurities?
- Who would be the lead organization?
- What other members would you invite?
- How would you address the issue?

Chapter Activity 3

Do a web quest and search for Community Coalitions. Write down what you have found. Identify how the established coalition reflects the stages of the Community Coalition Action Theory. Share your findings with your colleagues.

References

Allen, J., Dyas, J., & Jones, M. (2004). Building consensus in health care: A guide to using the nominal group technique. *British Journal of Community Nursing, 9*(3), 110–114.

Ansari, W. E., & Phillips, C. J. (2001). Interprofessional collaboration: A stakeholder approach to evaluation of voluntary participation in community partnerships. *Journal of Interprofessional Care, 15*(4), 351–368.

Atkins, S., & Murphy, K. (1993). Reflection: A review of the literature. *Journal of Advanced Practice, 18*, 1188–1192.

Berkowitz, B., & Wolff, T. (2000). *The spirit of the coalition.* Washington, DC: The American Public Health Association.

Butterfoss, F. D. (2007). *Coalitions and partnerships in community health.* San Francisco, CA: John Wiley & Sons, Inc.

Butterfoss, F. D., & Kegler, M. C. (2009). The community coalition action theory. In R. J. Di Clemente, R. A. Crosby, & M. C. Kegler (Eds.), *Emerging theories in health promotion practice and research* (pp. 237–276). San Francisco, CA: Jossey-Bass.

Center for Prevention Research and Development. (2006). *Evidence-based practices for effective community coalitions.* Champaign, IL: Center for Prevention Research and Development, Institute of Government and Public Affairs, University of Illinois.

Cohen, L., Baer, N., & Satterwhite, P. (2002). *Developing effective coalitions: An eight step guide.* Retrieved from http://www.preventioninstitute.org/index.php?option =com_jlibrary&view=article&id=104&Itemid=127

Feighery, E., & Rogers, T. (1990). *How-to guides on community health promotion: Guide 12. Building and maintaining effective coalitions.* Palo Alto, CA: Stanford Health Promotion Resource Center.

Florin, P., Mitchell, R., Stevenson, J., & Klein, I. (2000). Predicting intermediate outcomes for prevention coalitions: A developmental perspective. *Evaluation & Program Planning, 23*(3), 341–346.

Foley, E. (1915). Department of visiting nursing and social welfare: Vacation sketches. *American Journal of Nursing, 15*(6), 500–503.

Foster-Fishman, P. G., Berkowitz, S. L., Lounsbury, D. W., Jacobson, S., & Allen, N. A. (2001). Building collaborative capacity in community coalitions: A review and integrative framework. *American Journal of Community Psychology, 29*(2), 241–261.

Gabriel, R. M. (2000). Methodological challenges in evaluating community partnerships & coalitions: Still crazy after all these years. *Journal of Community Psychology, 28*(3), 339–352.

Goodkind, J. R., Ross-Toledo, K., John, S., Hall, J. L., Ross, L., Freeland, L., Coletta, E., & Becenti-Fundark, T. (2011). Rebuilding trust: A community, multiagency, state, and university partnership to improve behavioral health care for American Indian youth, their families, and communities. *Journal of Community Psychology, 39*(4), 452–477.

Greitemeyer, T., Schulz-Hardt, S., Brodbeck, F., & Frey, D. (2006). Information sampling and group decision-making: The effects of an advocacy decision procedure and task experience. *Journal of Experimental Psychology: Applied*, *22*(1), 31–42.

Hain, D. J., & Sandy, D. (2013). Partners in care: Patient empowerment through shared decision-making. *Nephrology Nursing Journal*, *40*(2), 153–157.

Kang, R. (1997). Building community capacity for health promotion: A challenge for public health nurses. In B. W. Spradley & J. A. Allender (Eds.), *Readings in community health nursing* (pp. 221–241). New York: Lippincott.

Kaye, G., & Wolff, T. (Eds.). (2002). *From the ground up: A workbook on coalition building & community development*. Amherst, MA: AHEC/Community Partners, Inc.

Linowski, S. A., & DiFulvio, G. T. (2012). Mobilizing for change: A case study of a campus and community coalition to reduce high-risk drinking. *Journal of Community Health*, *37*(3), 685–693.

Michaels, C. L. (2002). Circle communication: An old form of communication useful for 21st century leadership. *Nursing Administration Quarterly*, *26*(5), 1–10.

Nelson, G., Prilleltensky, I., & MacGillivary, H. (2001). Building value-based partnerships: Toward solidarity with oppressed groups. *American Journal of Community Psychology*, *29*(5), 649–677.

Porter-O'Grady, T., & Malloch, K. (2011). *Quantum leadership: Advancing innovation, transforming health care* (3rd ed.). Burlington, MA: Jones & Bartlett Learning.

Pressley, J. C., Barlow, B., Durkin, M., Jacko, S. A., Dominguez, D. R., & Johnson, L. (2005). *Journal of Urban Health*, *82*(3), 389–401.

Schön, D. (2006). *The reflective practitioner: How professionals think in action*. Aldershot, England: Ashgate Publishing Limited.

Soleimanpour, S., Brindis, C., Geierstanger, S., Kandawalla, S., & Kurlaender, T. (2008). Incorporating youth-led community participatory research into school health center programs and policies. *Public Health Reports*, *123*(6), 709–716.

Sullivan, T. J. (1998). Coalition building among diverse organizations: Concept analysis and model or theory design. In T. J. Sullivan (Ed.), *Collaboration a health care imperative* (pp. 253–300). New York: McGraw-Hill.

Truglio-Londrigan, M. (2013). Shared decision-making in home-care from the nurse's perspective: Sitting at the kitchen table—A qualitative descriptive study. *Journal of Clinical Nursing*, *22*(19–20), 2883–2895.

Truglio-Londrigan, M. (in press a). The patient experience of shared decision-making: A qualitative descriptive study. *Journal of Infusion Nursing*.

Truglio-Londrigan, M. (in press b). Practicing through a shared decision-making lens. *MEDSURG Nursing*.

Truglio-Londrigan, M., & Barnes, C. (2015). Working together: Shared decision-making. In S. B. Lewenson & M. Truglio-Londrigan (Eds.), *Decision-making in nursing: Thoughtful approaches for leadership* (pp. 141–162), Burlington: MA: Jones & Bartlett Learning.

U.S. Department of Health and Human Services. (2010). *Healthy People 2020*. Retrieved from http://www.healthypeople.gov/2010/state/toolkit/08partners 2002.pdf?visit=1

Vaughn, N. A., Jacoby, S. F., Williams, T., Guerra, T., Thomas, N. A., & Richmond, T. S. (2013). Digital animation as a method to disseminate research findings to the community using a community-based participatory approach. *American Journal of Community Psychology, 51*(102), 30–42.

Woehrle, L. M. (2003). Claims-making and consensus in collective group processes. In P. G. Coy (Ed.), *Consensus decision-making, Northern Ireland and indigenous movements* (*Vol. 24*, pp. 3–30). St. Louis, MO: Elsevier Science Ltd.

World Health Organization. (1978). *Declaration of Alma-Ata*. Retrieved from http://www.who.int/publications/almaata_declaration_en.pdf?ua=1

Chapter **7**

"I Told Them, Leave It Alone; It's OUR Center": Advocacy and Activism in Primary Health Care

Linda Maldonado

Chapter Objectives

By the end of this chapter, you will be able to:

1. Explore the role political advocacy plays within a primary health care framework.
2. Discuss the historical role of nurse-midwifery in shaping the policies and advocacy alliances in primary health care.
3. Discuss how midwifes politically advocate within social and racial diverse communities of women, children, and families.

Introduction

Political advocacy resonates within the philosophical framework of primary health care. This chapter uses the legacy of midwifery in the United States, focused mainly on the work of nurse-midwife Ruth Lubic, to explore the multiplicity of methods used in advocating for reductions in infant mortality in the latter part of the 20th century to the present. The methods of Lubic and her colleague Kitty Ernst, as well as other midwives, utilized grassroots activism that sought alternative methods toward change and improvement of infant mortality rates. Activist midwives formed intersectoral collaborative relationships in the 1970s and 1980s with social workers, community activists, physicians, nurses, and public health workers. Their work was effective because of a commitment to engage with members of the communities they served to develop processes of self-empowerment and education. Negotiating with the numerous stakeholders including hospital administrators and powerful physician groups such as the American College of Obstetricians and Gynecologists (ACOG) as well as the American Academy of Pediatrics, these activists were able to improve substandard medical and institutional treatment of marginalized pregnant women while pushing for alternative deliveries of obstetrical care that included the integration of nurse-midwives. Refusing to accept poverty as a major determinant of infant mortality within marginalized populations of women, nurse-midwives harnessed momentum from the growing women's health movement as well as the civil rights movement to bring a renewed sense of empowerment and democratization to birth. Through their work in neighborhoods blighted by poverty, nurse-midwives and their collaborative partners were able to improve the consistency of prenatal care by building strong networks of advocacy and social support. As a result, communities became engaged in their health care, effecting positive change in the health of pregnant women and infants. Today, despite lower infant mortality rates than a few decades earlier, Black women, regardless of socioeconomic status, still have higher rates of infant mortality than other racial groups. The history of nurse-midwives and health activists provides critical accounts that illuminate the evolutionary role of the nurse advocate in transforming communities. Furthermore, a historical understanding of successful nurse activist models such as the ones used by Lubic is essential as the United States continues to reform health care and expands the role of nurses in order to improve access to care.

Birthing Centers: Transforming 20th-Century Health Care

The history of Ruth Lubic's advocacy has its origins in her long relationship with the Maternity Center Association (MCA) in New York City. Founded in the early 1900s as a progressive era response to both Manhattan's and the nation's growing issues with maternal and infant mortality rates, the MCA pioneered an agenda for women and infants in several trendsetting ways. In the 1930s, the Lobenstine Clinic and School opened as one of the first in the nation to educate "a new and uniquely American practitioner—the nurse-midwife" (MCA, Box 1, Folder 9). In the mid- to late 1940s, MCA responded to postwar prosperity and decline in infant and maternal deaths through a new venue. By advocating for birth as a more satisfying event for the entire family, MCA situated itself as one of the initial proponents of the natural birth movement. However, the urban North was not the only geographic location where nurse-midwives were assessing maternal/child issues and entering into new avenues of health care delivery. The need to provide contextualized care for childbearing women and families was occurring in other parts of the country as well.

The rural South in the early 20th century witnessed different challenges, largely due to geographic and economic differences as compared to the urban North. In addition, mountainous areas such as the Appalachia in eastern Kentucky made health care difficult if not impossible for impoverished childbearing women and their families. Based upon her observations and studies of midwifery in Scotland, Mary Breckinridge started the Frontier Nursing Service (FNS) in 1925 (Goan, 2008). Established as a private charitable organization, FNS provided professional health care to women in the rural Appalachia of eastern Kentucky. Despite physician-led campaigns against midwives, Breckinridge proved that nurse-midwives could provide adequate maternity care to women and support the health care needs of the families. In the areas Breckinridge and her midwives served, maternal and infant deaths decreased dramatically (Goan, 2008).

Later in the 1940s, the Medical Mission Sisters, whose international work was limited during World War II, established a birthing center in Santa Fe, New Mexico (Cockerham & Keeling, 2010). Influenced by the progressive era's attention to reducing maternal-infant disparities as well as the success of both the FNS and MCA in providing health services to underserved populations, the Sisters focused on the dire situation in New Mexico. The Catholic Maternity Institute (CMI) served women of mostly Spanish American descent as well as trained both lay people and Catholic Medical Mission Sisters to become nurse-midwives. The Sisters advocated for and preferred their constituency to deliver at home and as such became another model alongside MCA for successful out-of-hospital birth. Despite CMI's successes, persistent struggles over finances eventually forced its closing in 1969 (Cockerham & Keeling, 2010).

The Lubic Method

The 20th-century history of nurse-midwifery reveals primary health care themes inherent to the negotiations nurse-midwives performed to both enter and serve their communities. These themes are (1) assess the community's needs and desires, (2) develop trusting relationships within the community, and (3) situate the community's needs before those of other stakeholders. Ruth Watson Lubic is no exception to her predecessors. Like those before her, Lubic situated herself within a community of women with a type of health care that delivered what the women and their partners were seeking and, in other cases, what the community needed to improve birth outcomes.

Early Years

The second of two children of John Russell Watson and Lillian (Kraft) Watson, Lubic was born Ruth Watson on January 18, 1927, in Bristol, Pennsylvania. Her father, a pharmacist, owned a drugstore, which he managed with the assistance of his wife. After the onset of the Depression, many townspeople and area farmers became too poor to pay for the services of a physician, and they would come to "Doc" Watson with their medical problems. He gave many of them pharmaceuticals on credit and often had to take out loans to replenish his stock. "If you were sick and needy, he tried to help" (Lubic, 1988).

In 1952, at age 25, having saved enough money to cover tuition and expenses, Lubic entered the School of Nursing at the Hospital of the University of Pennsylvania (Graham, 1996). As required of all nursing students at the time, Lubic spent 44 hours each week on duty at the hospital. In her tour as the evening charge nurse on a surgical ward, she ministered to patients who had undergone serious operations just hours before. Today, under policies now considered standard, these patients would have remained in recovery rooms or intensive-care units. "I marvel that I didn't run in terror," she has said (Baer, 2000). She served as student body president and sought (to no avail) for a reduction in the workweek from 44 hours to 40 hours. She also digressed from the norm when, a few weeks before graduation, she married William Lubic, a recent graduate of the University of Pennsylvania Law School. Lubic's marriage was, in a sense, an example of her independent thinking; most schools of nursing at that time did not admit women who were married or pregnant. In June 1959, after 4 years of marriage and 2 weeks after earning her BS degree in nursing, she gave birth to her son. Her husband witnessed the event, thanks to her obstetrician, who, in an action highly unusual for the time, made it possible for him to be present in the delivery room and to remain there with her and their newborn for an hour after the birth. Lubic's obstetrician, in another highly unusual action, convinced her to seek a degree in nurse-midwifery. Lubic applied and was accepted into the certificate program in nurse-midwifery at the MCA in 1961 (Lubic, 1988).

A 1956 editorial in the *American Journal of Obstetrics and Gynecology* reveals that there was some physician support for midwifery training based on MCA's positive reputation of educating and training midwives. The author, Dr. Herbert Thomas, speaks of a "continuing shortage of doctors" and "more than four million women who will need obstetrical care in the next and in succeeding year" (Thomas, 1956). With more than 7,000 births a year, its obstetrical service was one of the busiest in the nation. Lubic said that among the most valuable lessons she learned there was the importance of listening to and involving the whole family in decision-making about care, rather than having them stand by as passive recipients. She earned a certificate from MCA and the State University of New York in 1962. Upon completion of her nurse-midwifery education, Lubic immediately became an active participant in her professional organization by becoming the 331st member of the small but active American College of Nurse-Midwifery (ACNM). By the end of the year, Lubic was a member of the Program Committee and a year later became the Chair of Local Chapters. Involvement in her community of peers was rapid, and Lubic was elected vice president of the ACNM in 1964 (Baer, 2000).

Between 1963 and 1967, she worked as an MCA parent educator and counselor, a job in which she enjoyed seeing "apprehensive expectant couples change into confident families." Her satisfaction was tempered by the realization that her limited knowledge of different cultures was preventing her from responding adequately to the needs of some of her clients. As part of her early training as a midwife in MCA's certificate program, Lubic participated in home visits to postpartum women 24 hours postdelivery. Lubic recalled her home visit to a Puerto Rican young mother in East Harlem and the difficulties this young mother experienced as the result of language and cultural barriers. The national push to breastfeed was not a priority in the 1960s, and mothers were routinely taught how to prepare formula to feed their infants before hospital discharge. The infant formula at the time consisted of water, Karo syrup, and evaporated milk. Women were taught to make the formula, then sterilize the bottles on a stove. As Lubic recalled, for women who hardly spoke English and who did not have adequate income, these tasks could seem overwhelming and confusing (Lubic & Maldonado, 2009).

A Change Agent
In March 1970, Lubic was named the general director of the MCA. She assumed that position during a period when growing numbers of young American childbearing couples were becoming more knowledgeable about themselves, their reproductive systems, and health care. The 1970s was also a decade that witnessed the stunning loss of confidence many Americans held in the medical profession (Starr, 1982). The intersection of several major sociopolitical movements that included women's health provided a powerful context for Lubic's ideas surrounding women and birth. Lubic and her MCA board of directors felt the time was ripe to open an out-of-hospital birthing center for New York couples who desired more autonomy and control in their birth experiences (Lubic & Maldonado, 2009). At that time in New York City, many pregnant women were giving birth in their homes with no assistance from medical professionals. Lubic and her board of

directors knew an out-of-hospital center was safer than "do-it-yourself" homebirth and could also provide an empowering alternative to the traditional and technologically driven medical model of birth occurring in hospitals.

The Upper East Side Childbearing Center

The Childbearing Center (CbC) was established in a townhouse on the Upper East Side of the New York City borough of Manhattan in 1975. It was designed to offer comprehensive care in a homelike atmosphere to healthy families anticipating a normal birth experience. The CbC was established as a response to middle-class women in the late 20th century who wanted an interactive experience in health care and childbirth. As Lubic wrote, "It is a maxi-home and not a mini hospital. Actually our starting point was the home with all of the emotional support, comfort, and security that it offers" (Graham, 1996).

To help parents prepare for the responsibilities of child care, in 1978 the MCA added classes in "self-help education" to its program. In these classes the prospective mother was taught, among other things, to record her weight and test her urine regularly, and the father or other support person learned skills such as blood-pressure estimation and abdominal palpation. If, after checking the woman's records, the family's nurse-midwife detected any deviations from the norm, she would alert a staff physician. Clients received additional instruction in nutrition and physiological phenomena associated with pregnancy and birth. They also learned relaxation techniques to control tension and pain during labor and delivery. In addition, the center offered gynecological care as well as counseling in nutrition, reproduction, and sexually transmitted diseases. In an effort to foster emotional support, the CbC welcomed the presence of husbands, parents, and friends of the pregnant woman during the labor and delivery process. In another pioneering move, in 1979 the center began to offer classes to prepare children for the birth of siblings as part of its prenatal education program to ensure sibling bonding.

The comforts offered by the CbC stood in stark contrast to the sterile environments that pregnant women often encountered in hospital settings. For example, at the CbC there was a cozy family room and outdoor garden for women in labor and their companions as well as a kitchen where people could prepare a celebratory meal after the birth. At the CbC, mothers delivered their babies comfortably in a bed or in any other position they desired. The women giving birth at the CbC did not have to undergo continuous electronic fetal monitoring, and they rarely received anesthetics.

Lubic's CbC provided a fundamental change to how couples were treated during prenatal care, birth, and the postpartum period. For instance, mothers typically left the center within 12 hours of giving birth compared to the 24-hour stay in hospitals. CbC clients returned to their homes armed with information about normal postnatal recovery and infant care, and were given thorough follow-up care that consisted of a public health nurse visiting the family at home. New mothers also returned to the CbC for two postnatal examinations. The cost for these services was substantially lower than the charges for traditional obstetrical care in a hospital setting.

Lubic held onto her beliefs that providers of maternity care were not providing the services that their clients desired. In a 1972 article entitled "What the Lay Person Expects of Maternity Care: Are We Meeting These Expectations?" Lubic challenges the readers with these questions: Who are the laity and do all groups define maternity care the same way? (Lubic, 1972). Based upon data from MCA interviews, the majority of women and their partners felt that most providers of maternity care were not providing pregnant women and their partners with the care they desire. Despite a nod of approval from women's health and birth activists, Lubic's vision of creating an autonomous and empowering context for expectant couples was not well received by all.

The CbC generated much controversy in the medical community due its rising popularity with expectant New York City couples. Although couched in terms of concern for the safety of mothers and babies and the quality of care they would receive, the disapproval voiced by obstetricians and pediatricians was motivated primarily, Lubic eventually surmised, by fears of invasions into their professional territory and loss of power and income (Lubic, 1979). The CbC was becoming a competitor with obstetricians for the complete package of maternity care services with less cost to the pregnant couple as well as an experience that provided couples with the freedom they were not receiving in a hospital birth context. Another point of contention was the fact that Lubic hired certified nurse-midwives and physicians in a ratio of about 3 to 1 (Lubic, 1979).

The types of attacks Lubic endured varied from the ideological to the highly personal. Outlined in her dissertation, Lubic gave detailed descriptions of actions attributed to the CbC's detractors, ranging from multiple physician resignations from the MCA's Medical Advisory Board to discrediting the CbC with insurers, foundations, nursing students, as well as CbC birth families. In one account, Lubic and MCA board member Phyllis Farley attended a November 11, 1976, American Public Health Association convention. Farley felt she needed to accompany Lubic because "Ruth appears to be the focus of attack" and Farley felt her presence would emphasize the fact that the board is 100% behind the controversial Childbearing Center (Farley, 2011).

The Federal Trade Commission Weighs In

In 1981 the Federal Trade Commission conducted a study of the New York City obstetrical marketplace (Federal Trade Commission, 1981). The report found that New York City shared many characteristics with the national obstetrics market of the 1970s. For example, birthrates had declined considerably as hospital costs continued to rise. The trend in health planning was to consolidate underutilized obstetrics service, which meant closure entirely for smaller units. The study also asserted that projections of the birthrate made in the preceding decade had seriously underestimated the birthrate decline with the result that there was a surplus of obstetric professionals in certain markets.

Certain other characteristics of the obstetric market were also significant. First, New York City lost many middle-class residents in the 1960s due to the historical phenomena known as "white flight," and many young doctors followed them (Suarez, 1999). The result was that members of the medical establishment in New York City's prestigious medical schools were older and more conservative than their counterparts in comparable institutions elsewhere in the country. The consolidation of hospitals, particularly dramatic in the city, left more than 25 hospitals closed with more to be eliminated. Hospital closures left staff doctors looking for positions in other hospitals as well as limiting available training opportunities for residents and nurse-midwives. This created a heightened sense of competition for clients that MCA was attracting.

Such developments had serious implications for nurse-midwives generally and for the CbC specifically. According to one physician associated with a major New York City hospital and teaching center, the obstetric scene in the 1970s made obstetricians and nurse-midwives competitors for the low-risk births. This physician, a specialist in high-risk births and serious complications, envisioned a complementary relationship between low-risk pregnancies and births managed primarily by certified nurse-midwives with obstetric consultation as needed, leaving obstetricians and neonatologists (and hospital beds) available for the management of high-risk pregnancies, complicated deliveries, and newborns in need of intensive pediatric care. Because of the large number of skilled professionals competing for a limited number of low-risk mothers, the ideal utilization of obstetric resources had been delayed because many obstetricians were unwilling to relinquish the low risk-mother, the obstetrician's "bread and butter" (Federal Trade Commission, 1981).

Notwithstanding intense criticism from many doctors, within a short time facilities based on the model of the CbC began opening elsewhere. By the end of the 1970s, the CbC model prompted profound changes within New York City hospitals as well as influenced practice trends in obstetric care. Many of the major city hospitals were attempting to embrace a family-centered, maternity-care approach through expanded roles for nurse-midwives. In an effort to appeal to the low-risk mother, medical administrators pushed toward the incorporation of birthing rooms, increased support for breast-feeding and rooming-in, and shortened hospital stays for most mothers. The report summarized that the Childbearing Center modeled safe, family-centered care. The CbC also demonstrated a new cooperative model between physicians and nurse-midwives that directly benefitted low-risk mothers and their families (Federal Trade Commission, 1981).

Lessons Learned

In 1988, Lubic wrote for *Nursing Outlook* about her experiences with medical opposition and warned nurses to be on guard for overt and covert professional conflict as well as to be mindful of the true reasons behind opposition (Lubic, 1988). Lubic shared guiding principles, such as careful selection of colleagues and focusing on specific patient needs, that reflected much of her own professional experiences and tensions she endured while bringing her innovations to fruition. She also emphasized maintaining a sense of humor, and importantly, being proud of being a nurse. The CbC was representative of Lubic's political desire to bring increased autonomy to childbearing families. In this way, Lubic positioned her ideas as a challenge to medicine's hierarchical relationships. The CbC brought care beyond the geographic and political confines of the hospital space and its physician-nurse-patient relationships. She argued the CbC was an innovative response to the frustrations experienced by many women with hospital systems' depersonalized and routinized care centered on the medical model. Lubic's innovation brought not only a solution but an alternative care provider to the scene: the nurse-midwife. The care provided by midwives in the CbC was seen as empowering to families and comparably less expensive than a hospital birth (Fairman, 2010).

Another important component of Lubic's innovation was her call to professionals to critically examine the various kinds of women's social support before, during, and after birth. Lubic's interest in social support and how a birth center can provide this context to other groups of women served as the impetus for her next project in the South Bronx. She pondered over the important and still relevant question of just *who* are these women and families for whom providers deliver care? What are their national origins, gender, ethnicity, occupation, race, and age? How does culture affect their expectations? The answers heavily contribute to the type of care the woman and her support system will receive both from medical/hospital and midwifery/birth center models alike (Lubic, 1972). She drove home the argument of the importance of contextualized social support and medical care for the diverse types of childbearing women and their families.

The difference in outcomes of different paradigms of care is especially visible when attention is placed on minority and low-income women and their communities. As minority activist voices within the women's health movement declared, there are wide ravines of difference in terms of race and class when it comes to these various women's health needs, concerns, and expectations (Davis, 1983). These differences are embedded within the sociopolitical contexts from which these women emerge. Lubic (1972) argued that part of the foundation, in terms of care provided to women of various races and classes, must include measures to honor human dignity as well as assist in fostering a sense of personal worth.

Childbearing Center of Morris Heights

By 1983, the MCA's freestanding birth center became a model for others across the United States, with 103 out-of-hospital facilities in 30 states. Intent on demonstrating how a community-focused, empowerment-driven environment can positively affect change within marginalized communities, Lubic and the MCA embarked on another birth center project in the late 1980s. The location of the center contrasted with the middle-class homogeneity of the Upper East Side. With the second-worst infant outcomes in the nation, the South Bronx in the 1980s was particularly economically depressed with over 70% of residents living below the 200% federal poverty level. In addition, the percentage of Medicaid-insured residents was at 28.7%, and 33% were estimated to be uninsured. The racial composition of the area consisted of mostly Blacks and Hispanics.

The Childbearing Center of Morris Heights in the South Bronx opened in 1988. By utilizing the same type of philosophy that underpinned the Upper East Side's CbC, Lubic and her staff of midwives worked with the same goals of delivering innovative care within an environment that fostered ongoing education and social support delivered this time to a low-income minority community. As opposed to the context of White middle- and upper-class women, Lubic's Childbearing Center of Morris Heights fostered the opportunity for low-income women to "own" their care (Maternity Center Association & Wells, 1975). Lubic established care for a community whose concerns revolved around the barriers to care and high rates of infant mortality. Unsatisfied with the gap between provider and minority patient, Lubic sought ways to assist in the self-empowerment of minority and low-income women by teaching them to record their blood pressure, weight, and other prenatal measurements in their own medical charts. The women felt a sense of empowerment they had not experienced before in terms of their own health.

Lubic's work created within her a new understanding of the term "high-risk" childbearing. Through an intersectoral collaborative team approach with the women and families in their context and communities, Lubic and her team of midwives made an important discovery. By engaging women in their prenatal care, families as a whole became empowered, and birth outcomes began to slowly and steadily improve. The processes of assisting familial and community empowerment became an important part of understanding the puzzle of infant mortality within minority, low-income communities.

Lubic and her supporters offered a unique perspective for reforming health care. As women of economic means and influence, their philanthropic collaboration—as well as the politicization of the birth center and nurse-midwife movement—galvanized the larger women's health movement that occurred concurrently. The success and the message of Lubic's center spread and was viewed as a win for the national women's health movement as well as the expanding role of nurse-midwives.

The Family Health and Birth Center

The MCA's freestanding birth center became a model for others across the United States. By 1983, freestanding birth center care was being provided at 103 out-of-hospital facilities in 30 states. In 1996, according to the National Association of Childbearing Centers, now the American Association of Birth Centers (AABC), there were 145 birth centers in the United States and 100 more in various stages of development. The AABC estimated that there were 230 operating centers by 2011. The MCA and Maternity Care Coalition (MCC) remain key components of this system.

In 1993, Lubic became the recipient of a MacArthur Foundation Fellowship. Utilizing these award monies and other sources such as funding from HUD, Lubic subsidized her next project: the Family Health and Birth Center (FHBC) located in Washington, D.C. Lubic's center works with the collaboration of two other nonprofit service providers: the Healthy Babies Project (HBP) and Nation's Capital Child and Family Development. Following her own principles of working with communities and community leaders, Lubic engaged the interest of John Hechinger, a hardware magnate and owner of an abandoned Safeway supermarket. Hechinger, at first, was not interested in becoming a part of Lubic's plan, but he eventually donated the site to Lubic's project (Ly, 2007).

Similar to the Morris Heights CbC, the location of this endeavor was also in an impoverished area. Known as Ward 5 to D.C. planners and "Little Vietnam" to the local residents, the community had a reputation for high crime, poverty, and a grim statistic. The average life span of a man from Ward 5 was 56 years of age if he were lucky enough to survive the first year of life after birth (Lubic & Maldonado, 2009). In the 1990s, Ward 5, an area composed of primarily African Americans, held the nation's top spot for infant mortality and maternal disparities. Lubic recalled that in 1998, Ward 5's infant deaths were being reported as 25.1 per 1000 live births (Lubic & Maldonado, 2009). However, 2 years later, with the FHBC in operation, Ward 5's infant deaths dropped to 14 per 1,000 live births (See **Table 7-1**).

Before the physical structure was in place, Lubic believed she had to first gain trust from the community itself. As opposed to the Lower East Side CbC with its heterogeneous community comprised of several minority populations, Ward 5 was comprised of predominantly poor Blacks. Lubic and an African American employee from the Healthy Babies Project attended neighborhood community meetings. Once having gained entrance into the community, Lubic would show a video, *Hope Reborn: Empowering Families in the South Bronx* (Maternity Center Association & Wells, 1975).

Table 7-1

Indicators of Maternal Health, Child Health, and Mortality for the District of Columbia by Ward, 2000

Indicators	DC	Ward 1	Ward 2	Ward 3	Ward 4	Ward 5	Ward 6	Ward 7	Ward 8
Census Population 2000	572,059	80,014	82,845	79,566	71,393	66,548	65,457	64,704	61,532
Live Births Rate/1,000 pop	7,666 13.4	1,175 14.7	788 9.5	834 10.5	938 13.1	860 12.9	846 12.9	921 14.2	1,297 21.1
Births to Unmarried Women (Percent)	4,623 60.3	648 55.1	410 52.0	54 6.5	529 56.4	635 73.8	553 65.4	767 83.3	1,025 79.0
Births to Unmarried Women (Percent)									
Black	78.3	73.1	76.2	26.8	62.9	77.0	82.7	84.0	85.0
White	9.5	16.6	11.8	4.2	22.6	25.8	6.3	70.0	9.1
Hispanic	52.4	58.0	52.4	12.7	53.8	55.2	38.9	50.0	33.3
Births to Mothers <20 years (Percent)	1,086 14.2	139 11.8	99 12.6	6 0.7	115 12.3	155 18.0	138 16.3	184 20.0	250 19.3
Low Birth Weight Live Births[1] (Percent)	913 11.9	121 10.3	91 11.5	65 7.8	91 9.7	114 13.3	106 12.5	124 13.5	201 15.5
Low Birth Weight[1] to Teens <20 years (Percent)	117 10.8	19 13.7	12 12.1	1 16.7	7 6.1	15 9.7	15 10.9	18 9.8	30 12.0
Births with Adequate Prenatal Care (Percent)	65.1	70.0	63.8	81.9	70.0	64.5	63.5	59.1	53.4
Births with Prenatal Care Beginning First Trimester (Percent)	75.3	77.9	74.3	91.0	78.8	73.6	74.7	70.8	65.9
Infant Deaths (under I yr.) Rate (per 1,000 live births) [2]	91 11.9	11 9.4	6 7.6	1 1.2	5 5.3	12 14.0	17 20.1	16 17.4	23 17.7

[1]Low birth weight (under 2,500 grams or 5 lbs. 8 oz.).
[2]Due to the small number of infant deaths, infant mortality rates are highly variable and should be interpreted cautiously.
Source: State Center for Health Statistics Administration.

Reproduced from D.C. Department of Health and State Center for Health Statistics Administration. (2003). District of Columbia State Health Profile. Retrieved from http://doh.dc.gov/node/112742.

Lubic would also tell the participants in the meetings that she realized she was "the wrong color" and that she was from the "wrong place" (Lubic & Maldonado, 2009). Lubic also knew, similar to the support she had from her MCA board of directors; she needed the support of women leaders in this community.

In 1998, Veronica Hartsfeld, a member of the Carver Terrace neighborhood community, as well as president of the Carver Terrace Civic and

Tenants Association, met Ruth Lubic. As an advocate for her community members, Hartsfeld was also considered a respected and motherly figure for many of the community's Black youth. In an oral history interview with me, Lubic revealed that she knew she needed to make friends with Hartsfeld to gain the trust and acceptance of the community. Lubic, accompanied by a Black female employee of the Maternity Center Association, showed her 10-minute video of the Healthy Babies Project at community meetings organized by Hartsfeld. Largely as a result of the information shared and the approval of Hartsfeld, the community embraced Lubic's idea for a center (Lubic & Maldonado, 2009).

Hartsfeld, an established member of the community, was intimately familiar with her community's problems. Both Hartsfeld and Lubic relied on each other for the success of this program. Hartsfeld played an instrumental role toward her community eventually trusting Lubic and accepting the purpose of the health center. Indeed, the legacy of medical mistrust from Black communities undoubtedly played a significant role in the way Lubic approached the Carver Terrace community with the idea and philosophy of her birth center. Lubic recalled how she did not feel it was her choice to pick a color for the building when it was time to meet with painters. Lubic turned to the Carver Terrace community and asked them what color they wanted the building to be. With tears in her eyes, Lubic recalled the community women picked the color purple. When Lubic asked them why purple, they responded with, "because it is peaceful" (Lubic & Maldonado, 2009).

Lubic and Hartsfeld became friends despite their race and class differences within a geographic area that still held them apart. Hartsfeld had spent most of her life in the drug- infested community of Carver Terrace, whereas Lubic shared residences in New York City as well as Washington, D.C. They forged a bond because each had a vision of health care for women, and it was not what the general medical society was offering. As Hartsfeld was dying from breast cancer, Lubic visited her and shared with her that there was no graffiti or attempted break-ins to the center since its opening 3 years prior. Hartsfeld's answer to Lubic was, "I told them, leave it alone; it's OUR Center" (Lubic & Maldonado, 2009). These words provide a powerful glimpse into the intersectional nature and mutual ownership of a community center between women of various races and classes.

The bonds between the two women persisted for several years until Hartsfeld's death. Lubic and Hartsfeld's friendship is representative of the collaborative efforts of midwives' work with a wide range of women's health activists. Both women were leaders in their own sociopolitical contexts: one a well-known midwife, and the other, a highly respected member of an inner-city community. Their alliance as women creating positive change for other women became a powerful catalyst for community change.

Significantly, Lubic knew that if a midwife-led out-of-hospital birth center could make a difference in this location, the city of Washington, D.C., could stand to save millions of dollars in health care. The D.C. Center's positive birth outcomes and cost-effective services have saved the health care system $1,153,051 annually (Fairman, 2010). Other U.S. cities also had high rates of infant mortality, but choosing Washington, D.C., served an important roll in the various political implications of Lubic's work. The D.C. Center's midwives' positive birth outcomes were being displayed right under the eyes of those in the seat of government and in political power. She spent time on Capitol Hill delivering her message and providing policy changers and politicians with data and evidence to support the ongoing work of the nurse-midwife and nurse practitioner–led center.

The center's demographics also changed when in 2007 a birth center in Bethesda, Maryland, closed. Having served mostly privately insured patients, the clinic served a primarily White population. As a result of the closing, 30 some families came to look at Lubic's center. Some of those expectant mothers voiced concern that if they went into labor during the nighttime, they would have to enter the crime-ridden neighborhood where Lubic's D.C. center resides. Despite their concerns, many women from outside the Carver Terrace neighborhood do choose to deliver at the center (Lubic & Maldonado, 2009).

Through their work, Lubic and the nurse-midwives at the FHBC actualized cost savings and quality in a low-tech, high-touch environment that provided social support, careful monitoring during pregnancy and delivery, nutrition and health education, as well as community outreach. Lubic's individual advocacy and activism, her search for funding as well as consciousness raising has been foundational in her attempt to keep the FHBC independent from regulations that would distance nurse-midwives from the community they serve.

Discussion

In a recent interview by nurse midwife Andrea Sonenberg with Ruth Lubic and another pioneer nurse-midwife, Kitty Ernst, they spoke of their individual and collaborative work over the years. In 1983, Ernst and Lubic were the cofounders of the National Association of Childbearing Centers (NACC). Ernst went on to become the founder of the Community-Based Nurse-midwifery Education Project (CNEP) and is the Mary Breckinridge Chair of Midwifery at the Frontier School of Midwifery and Family Nursing (Osborne, Stone, & Ernst, 2005). Because of Ernst's work with midwifery education reform, students across the country are able to study to become nurse-midwives without leaving their homes and families for a long program of study. The long-term goal for CNEP is to increase the number of trained nurse-midwives across the country.

Both Lubic and Earnst have witnessed turmoil and triumph over their decades of work with women and birth. They have been friends for decades and have approached the democratization of birth and the advancement of midwifery from different vantage points: points that intersected while becoming strengthened by their complementary personalities and mutual respect (Lubic & Ernst, 2014). Much can be learned by examining the ways these women pushed the boundaries of health care and health care reform.

Predicated upon the work of Mary Breckinridge in the early 20th century and exemplary of the history of nurse-midwifery in the United States, both Lubic and Ernst became involved with policy and politics. Both women initially identified the particular needs of their community and population and followed that by applying innovative ideas to meet those needs. Success was dependent on collaboration with interagency and intersectorial support and novel use of resources. As Lubic's history reveals, navigating the waves of opposition from ideological opponents as well as competing stakeholders through advocacy and policy development is a foundational component to successful health care reform and primary health care. Networking with the community being served, building trust, and fostering the community's sense of ownership were also key components to Lubic's methods behind the politics of reform. Lubic's legacy of health reform also serves as the cornerstone to community reform. For Lubic, her desire to see communities gain the benefit of social support and nursing care still sits at an uncomfortable intersection with governmental regulation and medical models of birth.

Chapter Activities

1. How did MCC and Ruth Lubic's work shape the women's health movement going on at the time? How did Lubic and her organization navigate the social and political implications of their actions?

2. To what extent did the nature of the relationships within the Lubic's collaborative networks shape MCC's success and advocacy for maternal and infant care?

3. What does the democratization of health care mean to you in your own practice? Draw on the history of nurse-midwives in your response.

References

Baer, E. (2000). Trendsetter: Ruth Watson Lubic. *Journal of Obstetric, Gynecologic, & Neonatal Nursing*, 95–99.

Cockerham, A., & Keeling, A. (2010). Finance and faith at the catholic maternity institute, Santa Fe, New Mexico, 1944–1969. *Nursing History Review, 18,* 151–166.

Davis, A. (1983). *Women, race, and class.* New York: Vintage Books.

D.C. Department of Health. (2003). State Center for Health Statistics Administration. *Monograph: District of Columbia State Health Profile.* Washington, D.C.: Author.

Fairman, J. (2010). Go to Ruth's house: The social activism of Ruth Lubic and the family health and birth center. *Nursing History Review, 18,* 118–129.

Farley, P. (2011). *Farley interview.* Unpublished manuscript.

Federal Trade Commission. (1981). *Competition among health practitioners: The influence of the medical profession on the health manpower market, volume 11: The childbearing center case study.* Washington, DC: Federal Trade Commission.

Goan, M. B. (2008). *Mary Breckinridge: The frontier nursing service and rural health in Appalachia.* Chapel Hill: University of North Carolina Press.

Graham, J. (Ed.). (1996). *Current biography yearbook: 1991–1996.* New York: H. W. Wilson Company.

Lubic, R. W. (1972). What the lay person expects of maternity care: Are we meeting these expectations? *Journal of Obstetric, Gynecologic, & Neonatal Nursing, 1*(1), 25–31.

Lubic, R. W. (1979). *Barriers and conflict in maternity care innovation.* Doctoral Dissertation, Columbia University.

Lubic, R. W. (1988). Insights from life in the trenches. *Nursing Outlook, 36*(2), 62–65.

Lubic, R. W., & Ernst, K. (2014). *Interview by A. Sonenberg.* Unpublished oral history transcript developed for the Primary Health Care book.

Lubic, R., & Maldonado, L. (2009). *Interview with Ruth Lubic.* Unpublished manuscript.

Ly, P. (2007). A labor without end. *The Washington Post.* Published on May 27, 2007. Retrieved from http://www.washingtonpost.com/wp-dyn/content/article/2007/05/23/AR2007052301294.html

Maternity Center Association (Director), & Wells, P. (Producer). (1975). *Hope reborn: Empowering families South Bronx.* [Video/DVD]. The National League for Nursing.

MCA. (Box 1, Folder 9). *Lobenstine: The only school for nurse-midwives in the United States.* Unpublished manuscript.

Osborne, K., Stone, S., & Earnst, E. (2005). The development of the community-based nurse-midwifery education program: An innovation in distance learning. *Journal of Midwifery & Women's Health, 50,* 138–145.

Starr, P. (1982). *The social transformation of American medicine.* New York: Basic Books.

Suarez, R. (1999). *The old neighborhood: What we lost in the great suburban migration, 1966–1999.* New York: Free Press.

Thomas, H. (1956). A wider outlook in obstetrics. *American Journal of Obstetrics and Gynecology, 72*(6), 1305.

Chapter 8

Integrated Health Care Without Walls: Technology-Assisted Primary Health Care

Judith Lloyd Storfjell, Lucy N. Marion, and Emily Brigell

Chapter Objectives

By the end of this chapter, you will be able to:

1. Describe the determinants of health that place those with serious mental illness at great risk.

2. Examine how the "without walls" (WOW) initiative portrays care delivery from a primary health care perspective using a primary care point-of-service model.

3. Explore the role of technology in the enhancement of care access for this vulnerable population.

Introduction

Since 1998, the University of Illinois at Chicago College of Nursing (UIC CON), in collaboration with Thresholds, the leading freestanding psychiatric rehabilitation agency in Illinois, has provided integrated primary and mental health care to individuals with serious mental illness (SMI). A half-day clinic at one Thresholds site has evolved into three full-time nurse-managed health clinics called Integrated Health Care (IHC), which are a part of a Federally Qualified Health Center. The IHC clinics are staffed primarily by UIC CON faculty advanced practice nurses (APNs) with students at all degree levels. The APNs created an interprofessional team to provide integrated primary physical and mental health care services to people with SMI who are at risk of premature mortality from preventable illnesses, as well as other community residents in need of primary and/or mental health care. The IHC was supported by an active Community Advisory Committee with prominent Chicago citizens, including then Illinois State Senator and U.S. President Barack Obama and *New York Times* best-selling author Sara Paretsky.

IHC offers primary care with a point-of-care service model in the clinics, and all of the care is provided in the context of experiencing SMI while living in the community. Indeed, the development of IHC was more akin to *primary health care* as defined by the World Health Organization in the Declaration of Alma-Ata in 1978 and Nursing's Vision for Primary Health Care for the 21st Century (Marion, 1996). The IHC clinical team of UIC APNs and MDs and the Thresholds social services and mental health recovery teams together espoused this broader philosophical and holistic approach to health care. They addressed not only SMI combined with comorbid health conditions, but also the determinants of health that affect the overall well-being of the individuals served. The IHC and Thresholds interprofessional team members plus the many specialists and community service workers alternate leadership based on the individual's needs and location. The team members, in concordance with the person with SMI, participate in setting goals and actions to manage the challenges of mental illness, comorbid conditions, and the past experiences in a culture of cognitive dysfunction, poverty, violence, fear, loneliness, and often homelessness. Shared decision-making is inherent in the primary health care that leads to better health in this population.

IHC was built from the most fundamental elements of health care for a vulnerable population, developing new services as the individual and group needs unfurled. From the earliest screening health fairs, students and faculty identified the high use of hospital emergency departments for health care and the lack of access to any primary care services in the community. Public health nursing students assessed the community health of areas surrounding Thresholds group homes and identified pressing issues related to safe walking and other exercise availability, leading to physical activity intervention research (McDevitt, Braun, Noyes, Snyder, & Marion, 2005). From onsite care for young people in Thresholds's residential and community-based schools, the need for flexible health care emerged as the teens shifted on a dependent–autonomous continuum, and several creative, successful strategies were launched for the clinic and the school environment. When mothers in the Mother-Baby Program asked for services at that center, UIC IHC opened a clinic for mothers and children. Homeless care was delivered by IHC APNs directly to the individual in makeshift homes under bridges because the homeless staff specialists asked. After some years, the next reasonable step was to design and implement a telehealth program for hard-to-reach people where they lived in order to improve access, improve continuity of care, and obtain better outcomes.

This chapter describes how the IHC team advanced programming based on a primary health care approach with comprehensive, evidence-based integrated primary and mental health care and strategies to include services "without walls" (WOW) through telehealth technology.

The Population: Individuals with Serious Mental Illness (SMI)

About one half of Americans will have a mental disorder (DSM-5) sometime in their life, with first onset usually in childhood or adolescence. Prevalence of mental disorders for adults aged 18 or older in any one year is about 20% of the population, or 57 million individuals in the United States (DSM-5). As people with SMI experience higher levels of psychiatric symptoms, they are much more likely to have physical illnesses and become less able to manage their own health or access health care. Co-occurring conditions such as substance abuse, pregnancy, malnutrition, sedentary lifestyle, environmental exposures, violence, and accidental injury exacerbate general health problems. Moreover, some of these physical illnesses, including diabetes, can be caused or worsened by the very psychotropic medications that are effective in treating psychiatric symptoms.

Chronic mental illness is a "whole body condition" with a greater incidence of acute and chronic physical illnesses than is the norm, with documentation of differences in health risk, morbidity, and mortality going back many years (Kronick et al., 2009; Mitchell & Malone, 2006; Robson & Gray, 2007). In the schizophrenia trial of antipsychotic treatment effectiveness, Goff et al. (2005) found that subjects had significantly higher rates of smoking (68% vs. 35%), diabetes (13% vs. 3%), and hypertension (27% vs. 17%) as well as lower levels of HDL cholesterol (43.7 vs. 49.3 mg/dl), placing them at higher 10-year risk for coronary heart disease (9.4% vs. 7% in men; 6.3% vs. 4.2% in women) than the control group. In addition, higher rates of obesity are associated both with antipsychotics and other classes of psychotropics (Nardone & Snyder, 2014). People with SMI are also physically inactive, another health risk, and lack social contact (Daumit, Pratt, Crum, Powe, & Ford, 2002; Gibson, Carek, & Sullivan, 2011). General health is generally perceived as poor by those with SMI, as many suffer from obesity, lack of fitness, poor nutrition, high cholesterol, and smoking (Badger, McNiece, Bonham, Jacobson, & Glenberg, 2003). Poverty and the attending lack of transportation, adequate housing, and protection often add to the bleak picture of overall health status and poor quality of life.

On average, people with SMI die approximately 25 years earlier than those in the general population, in part due to excess suicides and accidents, but also due to excess deaths from the same *treatable comorbidities* that affect the general population, with the majority of premature deaths due to cardiovascular disease. In people with SMI, these comorbidities often go undiagnosed and untreated (Parks et al., 2006; Scharf et al., 2014). Although great strides have been made in delivering evidence-based primary care to the general population, patients living with SMI often have limited access to primary care and especially to care that competently addresses their special needs. Many outpatients diagnosed with schizophrenia and one or more other physical health problems, report difficulty receiving care. An analysis of Veterans Administration data showed that patients with a mental illness had fewer visits for medical care than patients without a mental illness, and the more severe the illness was, the fewer visits they had (Cradock-O'Leary, Young, Yano, Wang, & Lee, 2002). Young adults with schizophrenia and adults of all ages with bipolar disorder were least likely to receive medical care. Unfortunately, delays and underutilization of care can result in emergency room use and disproportionately high in-patient admissions for problems that are usually handled on an out-patient basis (Parks et al., 2006). Even when individuals with SMI do report utilization of general health services, they perceive barriers to accessing that care significantly more often than comparison groups (odds ratios > 3; Dickerson et al., 2003).

Typically delivery systems for mental health and physical health care are separate and often lead to significant inequalities both in access to care and quality of care, particularly for individuals of certain racial, ethnic, and socioeconomic status (Koyanagi, 2004). Often people with SMI are uninsured or insured through state Medicaid agencies. Health care providers are often reluctant to serve patients with Medicaid due to low reimbursement rates. The frequently co-occurring high rate of poverty is prevalent because most people with SMI are unable to work and are dependent on disability benefits. The benefits of integrating behavioral health and primary care is associated with better physical and behavioral health outcomes, reduced costs, and better patient experience of care (Blount et al., 2007; IHI 2014).

Description of Thresholds Members

Thresholds is Illinois's oldest and largest organization delivering services to people with SMI. For 50 years, Thresholds annually has served up to 7,000 people with SMI (called "members," reflecting the agency's beginnings as a clubhouse) with more than 100 program locations in the metropolitan Chicago area and Kankakee and McHenry counties. With its diverse array of services including psychiatric recovery-based rehabilitation, homeless outreach, housing, supported employment, independent living skill development, educational advancement, and mobile crisis services, Thresholds reaches an extremely vulnerable population—people with severe and persistent mental illness. Thresholds provide services in a host of area neighborhoods where access to other services is sometimes unavailable or difficult to obtain. As the agency's mission statement says, "Thresholds assists and inspires people with severe mental illnesses to reclaim their lives by providing the supports, skills, and the respectful encouragement that they need to achieve hopeful and successful future."

Many Thresholds members live on the South and West sides of Chicago, in high-crime, impoverished areas. Many of the areas in which Thresholds members live are recognized as "food deserts." In terms of health and health risk, Thresholds members unfortunately appear to fit the typical SMI profile. The most frequent primary care diagnoses for Thresholds member visits at IHC are type 2 diabetes (19%), hypertension (23%), tobacco abuse (17%), hyperlipidemia (14%), medication use (high-risk, long-term; 13%), general medical exam (11%), and asthma (5%).

Thirty-two percent of Thresholds members have a concurrent formal substance abuse diagnosis, 56% are African American, 43% are Caucasian, and 1% are Asian or Pacific Islander. Eight percent are Hispanic (ethnicity is in addition to race). Nearly two thirds of members are male (62% vs. 38%). Less than 1% are 20 years of age or younger, 16% are 20–29, 18% are 30–39, 31% are 40–49, 25% are 50–59, and 7% are 60 and older. The average level of education attained is 12 years, but it is important to note that up to 40% of members did not graduate from high school and, of these, 6% did not complete elementary school. It is equally important to note that high school graduation is not necessarily an indication of literacy; although formal studies are not available, there is a great deal of anecdotal evidence that some graduates of the Chicago Public School system are functionally illiterate. A pilot study of 30 Thresholds members, using the Newest Vital Sign tool (Weiss et al., 2005), found that 83% of members were in the low health literacy category compared to 69% in the general population of Chicago. A later master's student project ($n = 30$) identified that as many as 83% of IHC patients may have very low literacy. Virtually all Thresholds members have incomes that put them at or below the poverty level, although most members are assisted in accessing government benefits after they begin receiving Thresholds services (for some members this process can take years).

IHC History and Care Model

Recognizing these issues, IHC began in 1996 through collaboration between Thresholds and the UIC CON. Thresholds leaders envisioned a wellness goal for its members that included annual physical examinations and ongoing primary care. At the same time, a psychiatric/mental health nursing instructor and students from the UIC CON began to conduct health fairs and health education seminars at a Thresholds program site. They observed that Thresholds members could not access physical exams, much less comprehensive, continuing primary care. In response to the instructor's request to use FNP students to conduct physical exams, IHC was established.

By 1998, the APN faculty and students were conducting physical examinations and creatively adding to the Thresholds wellness objective by addressing the pressing need for ongoing primary and mental health care. These early services evolved into an academic nurse-managed center (IHC), embedding primary care services within Thresholds program locations to increase access to care. This model is termed "integrated care" because it brings primary care services to mental health treatment programs. However, the IHC model of care goes beyond providing primary care in Thresholds program locations. Because our nursing faculty are both primary care and mental health APNs, IHC integrates primary and mental health care, improving both physical and mental health outcomes (Blount et al., 2007; Davis et al., 2011; IHI, 2014). IHC clinicians collaborate extensively with the Thresholds clinical rehabilitation staff to ensure a fully integrated transdisciplinary care model.

However, this innovative service-delivery model goes further than simply providing primary care in mental health treatment settings. In this model, integrated care is the blending of concepts and processes of both mental and physical health care in the context of SMI and other comorbid diseases (McDevitt et al., 2005). For example, faculty family nurse practitioners (FNPs) provide primary care with additional psychotherapeutic knowledge and skills that may include cognitive-behavioral therapeutic methods, advanced psychopharmaco therapeutics, psycho education, and interventions for lifestyle change and self-care behavioral change. These FNPs bring an evidence-based community health care approach to the IHC team. Faculty IHC psychiatric/mental health advanced practice nurses (P/MH APNs) specialize in the delivery of psychotherapy and psychopharmaco therapeutics as well as the core APN skills of assessment and health monitoring of disorders classified as predominantly mental—to which they add knowledge of physical disorders. They are expert in group processes and in dealing with family conflicts. Some of the P/MH APNs prescribe psychotropic medications and conduct medication checks in collaboration with psychiatrists and FNPs.

The distinctive features of IHC are the cross training and creative planning for interventions that emerge and evolve regularly across both APN specialties through joint continuing education, grand rounds, case studies and mutual decision-making, consultation, and group leadership and member encounters. The "primary provider" for a member may change from FNP to P/MH APN based on the relationship and need of the member. All

IHC APNs participate in peer review, work closely with Thresholds case managers and psychiatrists, and refer members to medical and other specialists in the community.

A recent review of clinical outcomes 12 months after enrollment of IHC patients shows that:

- 70% had hemoglobin A1c (blood sugar laboratory test) levels below the national standard of 7, and 96% were below 9.
- 67% had LDL (bad cholesterol) levels less than the national standard of 100.
- 73% of hypertensive patients had blood pressures below 140/90 at their latest visit.
- 85% were vaccinated for influenza.
- 71% were vaccinated for pneumonia.
- 92% were vaccinated for tetanus.

IHC has received national recognition for its innovative model of integrated primary and mental health care, including the Illinois Nurses Association Innovation in Health Care Access Award in 2001, and the National Organization of Nurse Practitioner Faculties Faculty Practice Award for Excellence in Practice in 2003. In 2004, the Bazelon Center for Mental Health Law recognized IHC as one of four exemplars of primary care for people with mental illness. In 2008, the Agency for Healthcare Research and Quality (AHRQ) included IHC on the Innovations Exchange website, which recognizes innovative models of health care. In January 2011, IHC received an Excellence in Diabetes Management award from Your Healthcare Plus (YHP), the disease management division of Illinois Medicaid for achieving the best clinical outcomes in the state for patients with SMI. And in 2012, IHC was recognized by the American Academy of Nursing as an Edge Runner innovation.

The cornerstone of IHC service is an annual comprehensive health assessment received by each member. This assessment is comprehensive, integrates mental and physical best practices, and is individualized for each member. Faculty FNPs, all nationally certified and experienced in integrated health care, conduct the assessments. Members new to IHC, often with the assistance of their case manager, recount past and current illnesses, risks, and co-occurring conditions as well as past hospitalizations and surgeries, and provide a comprehensive health history. This process can be lengthy due to the member's abilities to recall and other cognitive deficits, and it may entail multiple requests for medical records and phone calls to past providers. When a member becomes comfortable and trusting enough with the clinicians to tolerate physical examinations, FNPs conduct comprehensive examinations that incorporate evidence-based screening, preventive measures, and diagnostic tests as needed.

Building on the comprehensive health assessments, IHC FNPs utilize evidence-based health management protocols they have developed especially for individuals with SMI, including flow sheets for medications, health indicators, and disease management. The disease management protocols are designed to integrate physical and mental health assessments and track member physical and mental health outcomes. Using these protocols as the basis, an individualized health plan (IHP) is created for each member. This IHP requires a session with active participation of the IHP team: FNP, member, Thresholds case manager, and, when indicated, other P/MH APN or mental health care providers. The session is a tailored, collaborative process in which members participate in discussions and decision-making until concordance among the participants is reached. The IHPs include disease management, wellness promotion, and the schedule for IHC follow-up visits.

Based on the health assessments and the collaborative planning sessions, IHPs may include participation in prevention programs such as smoking cessation, medication management, and weight reduction offering. The member-centered team identifies optimal expected outcomes and time frames according to context. Similar to the Thresholds rehabilitation management plans, these IHPs offer members a health contract to sign and take with them. The IHP is then implemented through follow-up visits and ongoing updating of progress and future plans. Continuing health assessment focuses on current health status, building on the information from previous visits, assessment of health indicators, and prevention of primary or secondary disease. In a review of multiples providers, the Institute for Healthcare Improvement (IHI, 2014) recently found that integrating behavioral health and primary care is associated with better physical and behavioral health outcomes, reduced costs, and better patient experience of care.

Quality assurance reviews indicate high rates of provider adherence to evidence-based practice guidelines and high-quality outcomes for members in our care. These outcomes are consistent with the literature that shows the quality of APNs (Lenz, Mundinger, Kane, Hopkins, & Lin, 2004). For example, analyses of our diabetes and dyslipidemia outcomes show improved systolic blood pressure and lipoproteins; analyses of provider adherence to hypertension and physical activity promotion guidelines show we consistently deliver recommended hypertension management and physical activity health promotion; and patient satisfaction scores are high.

These results are consistent with findings of recent RAND (Scharf et al., 2014) and Kaiser Family Foundation (2014) evaluations of integrated primary care and behavioral health programs, which found that health outcomes for consumers who received integrated services improved for diabetes, cholesterol, and hypertension, but not for obesity and smoking. RAND (Scharf et al., 2014) identified three features that were associated with greater consumer access to integrated services: co-location of services, integration of practices, and staff perceptions of belonging to a team. The Kaiser (2014) study identified five success factors: universal screening, navigators, co-location, health homes, and system-level integration of care, all of which have been included in the IHC model.

The Challenge

Although IHC had grown to three clinic sites, it was recognized in 2009 that IHC clinic-based services remained inaccessible for one group of Thresholds members—those who are homebound and socially isolated by limitations due to their serious mental and physical illnesses. Although IHC had made major inroads in reaching this extremely vulnerable population, a number of Threshold members still could not access primary care via IHC or other providers.

Adherence to recommended medications, activities, and appointments is critical for these high-risk individuals, yet IHC had a 35% clinic-visit "no-show" rate. This rate reflected some of the issues facing individuals with SMI: fear of health providers, forgetfulness due to cognitive limitations associated with medications and psychiatric disorders, and lack of resources to access transportation. Because of their multiple medical and psychiatric issues, these people may interact with numerous social and health care entities, often leading to fragmentation and confusion for the individual. Although IHC had made substantial penetration in providing services to Threshold members at the program sites where IHC clinics are located, outreach beyond our onsite clinic locations is still challenging. To increase access to these hard-to-reach individuals and deliver care where the people live, we sought Health Resources and Services Administration (HRSA) funding for technology to extend services that would not only increase access but would also dramatically increase adherence and support needed for necessary behavior changes.

Targeting the Need

The majority of Thresholds members who live in clustered housing (individual apartments in the same vicinity served by a Bridge center) or group homes live in areas of the Chicago Metropolitan Area that are designated as Health Provider Shortage Areas (HPSAs) or Medically Underserved Areas (MUA). Of these members residing in clustered housing and group home settings, fewer than 50% have an assigned primary care provider, and if they do, it is often their psychiatrist. It was therefore determined that IHC's initial telehealth intervention would be targeted at this underserved population.

The Telehealth Project

To improve clinical outcomes for this unique population, we decided to follow the recommendations of the President's New Freedom Commission (2003) and utilize innovative, cost-effective strategies to improve access and clinical outcomes for these hard-to-reach members. This approach would transcend IHC's clinic walls to dramatically improve our outreach through the use of telemonitoring technology, shown to increase access, adherence, and quality of care in hard-to-reach, vulnerable populations. Home tele-monitoring (HT) technology has become increasingly interactive, less expensive, standardized, and available. HT is the process of using remote computer equipment to monitor the condition of a patient, and relay information over a telephone line or wireless connection to a central site. Various sensing devices connected to the monitors can transmit a variety of physiological measures such as weight, pulse, blood pressure, respiration, pulse oximetry, and blood glucose readings (Tweed, 2003). HT allows clinicians to monitor parameters over time and frequently. In essence it is an alternative way and means for providers to enter into the community and gain access to their members.

As we planned this project, our review of the literature found that HT provides a means to keep unstable patients at home under close supervision, facilitating early detection of changes and intervention (Cherry, Dryden, Kobb, Hilsen, & Nedd, 2003; Storfjell et al., 2008), thus preventing many adverse events, even with less frequent onsite observation—especially critical for homebound patients (Louis, Turner, Gretton, Baksh, & Cleland, 2003). HT has also been used as a way to increase clinician productivity, thus reducing costs for high-risk patients (Ryan, Kobb, & Hilsen, 2003). Although telemonitoring was introduced into health care as a method for distance monitoring of clinically unstable individuals, its impact in changing behavior by constant reminders with immediate feedback can be extremely beneficial in focusing on an individual with SMI on a particular behavior critical to successful management of both mental and physical health.

Studies also found no difference in patient satisfaction between HT patients and traditional care patients, suggesting that patients do not perceive any lessening of care quality when using HT (Dansky & Bowles, 2002; Pare, Jaana, & Sicotte, 2007). In addition, usability by a variety of patients has been unexpectedly high. Several studies have reported that even the frail and elderly can use HT (Buckley, Tran, & Prandoni, 2004); that age was not a factor in the proficient use of monitors (Chetney, 2003); that patients had a high degree of readiness to adopt this new technology because of its potential to support independence; that patients perceived their health had improved in dimensions including pain, physical, and social functioning (Pare et al., 2007; Ryan et al., 2003); and that preventable hospitalizations were reduced (Jia, Chuang, Wu, Wang, & Chumbler, 2009). The clinical value of HT has been clearly demonstrated for unstable cardiovascular and diabetic patients—both in improving clinical outcomes and in reducing the need for emergent and in-patient care.

By adding HT to the IHC service delivery model, we hoped to gain access to Thresholds members unable to access our services, thereby advancing our model of integrated care. This innovative outreach program was referred to as Integrated Health Care Without Walls (IHC WOW). IHC WOW teamed IHC faculty FNPs with Thresholds case managers in "WOW

Continuity Teams" to ensure continuity of integrated health care across sites of care. Use of HT was expected to enhance both the efficiency and effectiveness of care, specifically targeted at improving adherence to medication regimes and lifestyle changes and to monitor clinical parameters of unstable members (e.g., those with diabetes, obesity, or cardiovascular disease). Funding was obtained from HRSA and the 3-year initial project was implemented in 2010.

Telemonitoring kiosks were placed in Thresholds group homes where a group of unstable diabetic and/or cardiovascular members resided or where there were several SMI members with obesity or medication-adherence problems. This technology supports the WOW model's "assess/monitor" intervention by using technology to monitor certain physical parameters more frequently in order to adjust treatment regimens in "real time," and to reinforce adherence to plans of care. Members were supported in using the monitors, which transmitted a variety of parameters (blood sugar, weight, blood pressure, pulse oximetry, heart rate) to a central IHC monitoring station and related database, allowing an IHC RN to monitor changes in clinical conditions and provide immediate reinforcement of medication, diet, and other lifestyle behaviors.

The Thresholds onsite resident manager was trained in the use of the telemonitoring equipment and assisted individual members to transmit their data (blood glucose, etc.). All measures were transmitted to a central IHC WOW location where individual member profiles were created. The location was immediately notified if a member was late in transmitting or if the results were outside the member's established parameters. An IHC WOW RN monitored the transmissions and contacted the group home staff person if a transmission was delayed, thus promoting consistency of reporting. The member's APN was notified if measures fell outside (above or below) the member's acceptable range. The APN or RN then contacted the member either by telephone or house call and made the necessary treatment adjustments.

HT Project Outcomes

In the first year of the grant, we determined there might be a need for individual monitors for members receiving house calls. Therefore, we secured both multiuser monitors and individual monitors. In the final year of the grant, telemonitoring expanded to 37 members in six group homes and one individual home. This expansion included a high-risk vulnerable subgroup in our population: hearing-impaired members who have significant cognitive impairment due to hearing loss and mental illness. These patients conducted 1,509 telemonitoring visits through year 3 of the grant.

Group homes conducted telemonitoring "visits" 3 times per week. The monitors collected and transmitted key biometric data such as weight, blood pressure, and blood glucose. The IHC nurse accessed and reviewed the results at the IHC clinic sites. The IHC nurse followed the IHC WOW telemonitoring protocol and consulted with the IHC APN as needed. The following reflects telemonitoring data analysis through year 3 of the HRSA project:

> **Weight**: 60% of obese members lost weight, 24% stabilized weight, and 16% gained weight. Stabilization of weight is a significant achievement in this population as psychiatric medications cause weight gain.
>
> **Blood pressure**: Three of four group homes evaluated in year 3 exceeded blood pressure targets: (1) in group home 1, 77% of the blood pressures were below the standard of 140/90; (2) in group home 2, 83%; in group home 3, 86%; and in group home 4, 69%.
>
> **Blood glucose**: 86% of the members with diabetes had blood sugars within the normal range and clinic A1c blood test results that met the American Diabetes Association standard, which exceeds our target of 75%.

In addition to these quantitative outcomes, the following qualitative results show telemonitoring to be a promising intervention for individuals with SMI. Two members' physical and health status improvement led to their recent transition from group to independent living. One of the members in independent living requested a telemonitor to support his continued efforts in weight loss. Another member with inconsistent blood pressure, glucose, and weight management, who is active in telemonitoring, attributes his successful smoking cessation to his increased focus on health during telemonitoring. Members in the initial telemonitoring pilot had rare clinic visits. After telemonitoring began, IHC RNs and APNs noted better adherence to clinic visits. The IHC staff identified several members with very high heart rates and referred them for cardiology evaluations. In addition, elevated blood pressures were managed with medication changes and clinic visits, mitigating complication risks.

The clinical targets were set based on a normal population. However, through this project, we have learned even more about how difficult it is to effect clinical changes in this very complex population. In fact, the dean of our College of Medicine, a psychiatrist, was amazed with the results we have achieved, calling them "remarkable." We have found that telemonitoring is an extremely effective tool for monitoring and affecting lifestyle changes for this very high-risk population.

Member Satisfaction

Focus groups measured telemonitoring satisfaction and were led by a UIC CON advanced community health student. The focus groups included the initial 12 members in the telemonitoring pilot group. The following questions were discussed in the focus groups: (1) what is your main problem, (2) what do you like about being monitored 3 times per week, (3) what don't you like about telemonitoring, (4) has it made any difference with your health (diet, blood pressure, diabetes), and (5) would you recommend it to your family? All of the members were able to identify a main health problem. The members were all very positive about the experience and did not have any negative responses. The members all believed that telemonitoring was improving their health and they would recommend it to family and friends.

Mental Health Status

Recovery from mental illness is a process of empowerment in which the individual develops personal, social, environmental, and spiritual connections that assist in overcoming the challenges of illness. The house call approach is member centered and allows the provider to (1) enter the everyday lives of people with SMI, and (2) understand the members' situations from their perspectives. In so doing, the provider enters into a partnership with the client. In collaboration with the case manager, who manages a long-standing relationship with the member, provider-member-case manager interaction provides the person with SMI socialization experiences and skills training for illness self-management where they live and at the level of intensity they can tolerate. Through outreach, comprehensive, accessible, and integrated services are made available in a graded stepwise manner.

Conclusion

IHC WOW, a project using telemonitoring health care service for people with SMI in their homes, was an innovation resulting directly from the primary health care and member-centered approach to designing and managing relevant health care for people, their families, and communities. After approximately 10 years of IHC activity, the UIC CON faculty and students identified the need for improved access and continuity of care through telemonitoring to gain better health outcomes. This project was "ahead of the curve." Nevertheless, the method was successful in terms of health outcomes, satisfaction to the client and other members of the extended health care team, and exploration of outreach strategies to people whose life expectancy and quality of life are curtailed by SMI. Based on the positive results, IHC began exploring other telehealth opportunities, including implementation of a virtual clinic. This study should be replicated with attention to "lessons learned" and the continuing need to identify ways to provide ever improved health care to this vulnerable population from a primary health care perspective.

Chapter Activities

This IHC WOW case study reflects challenges that people with serious mental illness overcame when accessing continuing and appropriate health care with telemonitoring visits. The report, however, reveals few of the obstacles faced by the dedicated and futuristic clinicians who delivered the care.

1. Discuss reported and probable other barriers to APN delivery of quality care delivery by the WOW program and possible ways to overcome these barriers.

2. Design a "virtual" system for people with serious mental illness, merging knowledge of the current explosion in home delivery of primary and mental health care and the WOW model.

3. Identify other process and outcome measures you would add to the IHC WOW service for validating the worth of the program, improving care, and marketing to possible funders.

4. Prepare "elevator speeches" to encourage people with SMI and group home staff to participate in WOW-type services.

5. Describe whom you would invite to serve on your advisory committee to help maximize telehealth for people with serious mental illness.

References

Badger, T., McNiece, C., Bonham, E., Jacobson, J., & Glenberg, A. (2003). Health outcomes for people with serious mental illness: A case study. *Perspectives in Psychiatric Care, 39*(1), 23–32.

Blount, A., Schoenbaum, J., Kathol, R., et al. (2007). The economics of behavioral health services in medical settings: A summary of the evidence. *Professional Psychology: Research and Practice, 38*(3), 290–297.

Buckley, K. M., Tran, B. O., & Prandoni, C. M. (2004, August 31). Receptiveness, use and acceptance of telehealth by caregivers of stroke patients in the home. *The Online Journal of Issues in Nursing, 9*(3), 9.

Cherry, J. C., Dryden, K., Kobb, R., Hilsen, P., & Nedd, N. (2003). Opening a window of opportunity through technology and coordination: A multisite case study. *Telemedicine Journal and e-Health, 9*(3), 265–271.

Chetney, R. (2003). Home care's challenge: Move the information…not the patient. *Home Healthcare Nurse, 21*(1), 712.

Cradock-O'Leary, J., Young, A., Yano, E., Wang, M., & Lee, M. (2002). Use of general medical services by VA patients with psychiatric disorders. *Psychiatric Service, 53*, 874–878.

Dansky, K. H., & Bowles, K. H. (2002). Lessons learned from a telehomecare project. *Caring, 11*, 18–22.

Daumit, G. L., Pratt, L. A., Crum, R. M., Powe, N. R., & Ford, D. E. (2002). Characteristics of primary care visits for individuals with severe mental illness in a national sample. *General Hospital Psychiatry, 24*, 391–395.

Davis, K. E., Brigell, E., Christiansen, K., Snyder, M., McDevitt, J., Forman, J., Storfjell, J. L., & Wilkniss, S. M. (2011). Integrated primary and mental health care services: An evolving partnership model. *Psychiatric Rehabilitation Journal, 34*(4), 317–320.

Dickerson, F. B., McNary, S. W., Brown, D. H., Kreyenbuhl, J., Goldberg, R. W., & Dixon, L. B. (2003). Somatic healthcare utilization among adults with serious mental illness who are receiving community psychiatric services. *Medical Care, 41*, 560–570.

Gibson, M., Carek, P. J., & Sullivan, B. (2011). Treatment of co-morbid mental illness in primary care: How to minimize weight gain, diabetes, and metabolic syndrome. *International Journal of Psychiatry Medicine, 41*(2), 127-1-42.

Goff, D. C., Cather, C., Evins, E., Henderson, D. C., Freudenreich, O., & Copeland, P. M. (2005). Medical morbidity and mortality in schizophrenia: Guidelines for psychiatrists. *Journal of Clinical Psychiatry, 66*, 183–194.

Institute for Healthcare Improvement. (2014, March). *IHI 90-day R&D project final summary report: Integrating behavioral health and primary care.* Cambridge, MA: Institute for Healthcare Improvement. Retrieved from www.ihi.org

Jia, H., Chuang, H., Wu, S. S., Wang, X., & Chumbler, N. R. (2009). Long-term effect of home telehealth services on preventable hospitalization use. *Journal of Rehabilitation Research & Development, 46*(5), 557–566.

Kaiser Family Foundation. (2014). *Integrating physical and behavioral health care: Promising Medicaid models.* Menlo Park, CA: The Kaiser Commission on Medicaid and the Uninsured.

Koyanagi, C. (2004). *Get it together: How to integrate physical and mental health care for people with serious mental disorders.* A Report by the Bazelon Center for

Mental Health Law. Retrieved from http://www.bazelon.org/LinkClick .aspx?fileticket=FamA0HBviIA=

Kronick, R. G., Bella, M., & Gilmer, T. P. (2009, October). *The faces of Medicaid III: Refining the portrait of people with multiple chronic conditions.* Center for Health Care Strategies. Retrieved from http://www.chcs.org/resource/the-faces-of-medicaid-iii-refining-the-portrait-of-people-with-multiple-chronic-conditions/

Lenz, E. R., Mundinger, M. O., Kane, R. L., Hopkins, S. C., & Lin, S. X. (2004). Primary care outcomes in patients treated by nurse practitioners or physicians: Two-year follow-up. *Medical Care Research and Review, 61,* 332–351.

Louis, A. A., Turner, T., Gretton, M., Baksh, A., & Cleland, J. G. F. (2003). A systematic review of telemonitoring for the management of heart failure. *European Journal of Heart Failure, 5,* 583–590.

Marion, L. (1996). *Nursing's vision for primary health care in the 21st century.* Washington, DC: American Nurses Association.

McDevitt, J., Braun, S., Noyes, M., Snyder, M., & Marion, L. (2005). Integrated primary and mental health care: Evaluating a nurse-managed center for clients with serious and persistent mental illness. *Nursing Clinics of North America, 40*(4), 779–790.

Mitchell, A. J., & Malone, D. (2006). Physical health and schizophrenia. *Current Opinion in Psychiatry, 19*(4), 432–437.

Nardone, M., & Snyder, S. (2014, February). *Integrating physical and behavioral health care: Promising Medicaid models.* Kaiser Commission on Medicaid and the Uninsured.

Pare, G., Jaana, M., & Sicotte, C. (2007). Systematic review of home telemonitoring for chronic diseases: The evidence base. *Journal of the American Medical Informatics Association, 14*(3), 269–277.

Parks, J., Svendsen, D., Singer, P., & Foti, M. E. (Eds.). (2006, October). *Mortality and morbidity in people with serious mental illness.* National Association of State Mental Health Program Directors. Retrieved from http://www.dsamh.utah. gov/docs/mortality-morbidity_nasmhpd.pdf

President's New Freedom Commission on Mental Health. (2003). *Achieving the promise: Transforming mental healthcare in America.* Retrieved from http:// govinfo.library.unt.edu/mentalhealthcommission/reports/FinalReport /downloads/FinalReport.pdf

Robson, D., & Gray, R. (2007). Serious mental illness and physical health problems: A discussion paper. *International Journal of Nursing Studies, 44*(3), 457–466.

Ryan, P., Kobb, R., & Hilsen, P. (2003). Making the right connection: Matching patients to technology. *Telemedicine Journal and e-Health, 9*(1), 81–88.

Scharf, D. M., Eberhart, N. K., Hackbarth, N. S., Horvitz-Lennon, M., Beckman, R., & Burnam M. A. (2014). *Evaluation of the SAMHSA Primary and Behavioral Health Care Integration (PBHCI) grant program: Final report (Task 13)* RR-546-DHHS. Santa Monica, CA: RAND Corporation. Retrieved from http://www.rand.org/pubs/research_reports/RR546.html

Storfjell, J. L., Brigell, E., Christiansen, K., McDevitt, J., Miller, A., Snyder, M., & Pavick, D. (2008, December). WOW specialty home care service for individuals with serious mental illness. *Home Health Care Management & Practice, 21*(1), 23–32.

Tweed, S. C. (2003). Seven performance-accelerating technologies that will shape the future of home care. *Home Healthcare Nurse, 21*(10), 647–650.

Weiss, B. D., Mays, M. Z., Martz, W., Castro, K. M., DeWalt, A., & Hale, F. A. (2005). Quick assessment of literacy in primary care: The newest vital sign. *Annals of Family Medicine, 3,* 514–522. doi: 10.1370/afm.405

Chapter 9

Global Nursing: Primary Health Care Perspective in Caring for Populations

Majeda M. El-Banna and Carol Lang

Chapter Objectives

By the end of this chapter, you will be able to:

1. Identify the current global disease burden and its projection by 2030.
2. Discuss the definitions of international health, public health, and global health.
3. Explore the relationship between primary health care and global nursing.
4. Discuss the educational requirement and competencies of the global nurse.
5. Appraise worldwide examples of nurses' primary health care initiatives.

Chapter Overview

This chapter introduces global nursing from a primary health care (PHC) perspective. The world in which we live is more interconnected today than ever before. Concepts of globalization and major health challenges in terms of global burden of disease are discussed as is the important contribution nurses make to global health in health promotion and disease prevention. PHC nurses need to focus on reducing global health problems by prioritizing current and emerging health needs and challenges and developing interprofessional collaborations that support and strengthen programs that promote health care for all. To achieve global health for all, a collaboration between countries worldwide is required. There is ample evidence that no country can protect the health of its citizens alone.

International Health, Public Health, Global Health, and Primary Health Care

The World Health Organization (WHO) is predominantly associated with the evolved term "global health" and played a role in transitioning from the use of international health or public health to global health. Global health is the emergent, preferred, fashionable, and increasingly used term (Brown, Cueto, & Fee, 2006); however, it is still used interchangeably with international health and public health (Khubchandani, 2012). International heath has a limited perspective, concentrating on disease control across the boundaries of nations (Brown et al., 2006). Since 2007, the world has been implementing International Health Regulations proposed in 2005 that aim at preventing, protecting against, controlling, and providing a public health response to the international spread of disease (WHO, 2015a). However, WHO (2015b) describes public health as "all organized measures (whether public or private) to prevent disease, promote health, and prolong life among the population as a whole. Its activities aim to provide conditions in which people can be healthy and focus on entire populations, not on individual patients or diseases." Public health focuses mainly on health promotion and disease prevention, whereas global health involves both preventive measures and curative care. There is no widely agreed definition for global health; for example, Koplan and colleagues (2009) defined global health as "an area for study, research, and practice that places a priority on improving health and achieving equity in health for all people worldwide. Global health emphasizes transnational health issues, determinants, and solutions; involves many disciplines within and beyond the health sciences and promotes interprofessional collaboration; and is a synthesis of population-based prevention with individual-level clinical care." This definition was adopted by the Expert Panel on Canada's Strategic Role in Global Health (Campbell, Pleic, & Connolly, 2012). To meet the needs of individuals, communities, populations, and countries, the Centers for Disease Control and

Prevention (CDC, 2014) has developed a global health strategy for the years 2012 to 2015 that is a systematic approach to global health. It advances four main global health goals: improving the health and well-being of people around the world; improving capabilities for preparing and responding to infectious diseases and emerging health threats; building country public health capacity; and maximizing organizational capacity. In addition to the concepts of international health, public health, and global health, all emphasized by the WHO, work centering on the philosophical belief of primary health care is at the very core of health for all. Many countries do accept this philosophical belief and strive to develop a framework that addresses the essential elements of primary health care that embraces health for all as a right; however, the provision of primary health care delivered by all levels of providers remains inadequate in many developing and developed countries (Rao & Pilot, 2014).

The Millennium Development Goals and Global Burden of Disease

The United Nations Millennium Development Goals (MDGs) were introduced in 2000. Some of these goals were specifically developed to reduce poverty, hunger, and disease by the year 2015. **Table 9-1** provides an overview of the MDGs that represent the holistic nature of primary health care. The MDGs are interdependent; all the MDGs influence health or are affected by health. For example, reducing poverty and hunger (MDG 1) positively influences and depends on better health (MDGs 4-6).

Progress toward the attainment of these goals is measured by the Institute for Health Metrics and Evaluation (IHME, 2015a), whose goal is to identify and to share data that depicts global health trends for the delivery of evidence-based information to policy makers, researchers, and funders for change. Specifically, within the IHME, the Global Burden of Disease

Table 9-1	
Millennium Development Goals (MDGs)	
Goal 1	Eradicate extreme poverty and hunger
Goal 2	Achieve universal primary education
Goal 3	Promote gender equality and empower women
Goal 4	Reduce child mortality
Goal 5	Improve maternal health
Goal 6	Combat HIV/AIDS, malaria, and other diseases
Goal 7	Ensure environmental sustainability
Goal 8	Develop a global partnership for development

Modified from The Millennium Development Goals Report, © 2015 United Nations.
http://www.un.org/millenniumgoals/2015_MDG_Report/pdf/MDG%202015%20rev%20(July%201).pdf page 72. Reprinted with the permission of the United Nations.

(GBD) presents and analyzes data to identify trends in health worldwide. The GBD provides information about risk factors related to disease, injury, and health outcomes for different demographic populations. It provides comparative information for countries on health progress and the potentially avoidable leading causes of health loss. Through this work, changing national trends can be identified and specific interventions to improve health care systems—locally, nationally, and internationally—can be planned and implemented (IHME, 2015b).

Global Progress Toward Health

A systematic analysis of the Global Burden of Disease Study in 2013 examined the progress made with regard to the MDGs, and some examples follow. The results related to MDG 4, "reduce child mortality," indicated that the global child mortality rate has decreased since 2003 at a faster rate than in the 1970s and 1980s as a result of increased development assistance for health. Deaths of children under 5 years old had dropped dramatically since 2000, especially in sub-Saharan Africa. The child mortality rate had decreased by almost 50% since 1990; 6 million fewer children died in 2012 than in 1990. However, the world is still falling short of the MDG child mortality target of a two-thirds mortality reduction, and only 27 developing countries are expected to achieve it. In 2013, 26 countries accounted for 80% of child deaths worldwide (Afghanistan, Angola, Bangladesh, Brazil, Burkina Faso, Cameroon, Chad, China, Cote d'Ivoire, Democratic Republic of the Congo, Ethiopia, Ghana, India, Indonesia, Kenya, Malawi, Mali, Mozambique, Niger, Nigeria, Pakistan, Philippines, Somalia, Sudan, Tanzania, and Uganda). Even though child mortality decreased significantly in India, Eastern Europe, and almost all countries in sub-Saharan Africa, the 10 countries with the highest under-5 mortality rate in 2013 were all in sub-Saharan Africa, and many countries in west and central Africa will still have high levels of under-5 mortality in 2030. The rate of decline in child mortality has slowed down, however, in many Latin America countries (United Nations, 2014; Wang et al., 2014).

Another systematic analysis that examined the progress of MDG 5, "improve maternal health," revealed that 300,000 women died globally in 2013 from causes related to pregnancy and childbirth. The proportion of deliveries in developing regions attended by skilled health personnel rose from 56% to 68% between 1990 and 2012. The global rate of maternal mortality has decreased by 1.3% per year since 1990. In 2013, 16 countries, including 7 developing countries, were expected to achieve the MDG 5 target of a 75% reduction in the maternal mortality rate by 2015. There were two trends in developing countries, one showing a decrease in the maternal mortality rate in Asia and Latin America and the other showing stagnation or increases in the maternal mortality rate in sub-Saharan Africa and Oceania from 1990 to 2003. Surprisingly, an increase in some high-income countries, such as the United States, went against the predicted maternal mortality rates (Kassebaum et al., 2014; United Nations, 2014). Similar to MGD 4, the Millennium Declaration in 2000 and increased development assistance contributed to progress in maternal, newborn, and child health.

The latest analysis from the Global Burden of Disease study in 2013 shows that since adoption of MDG 6, "combat HIV/AIDS, malaria and other diseases," by governments worldwide, the global burden and incidence rate of HIV/AIDS, malaria, and tuberculosis have decreased significantly. Antiretroviral medicines were delivered to 9.5 million people in developing regions in 2012. Malaria interventions saved the lives of 3 million young children between 2000 and 2012. Also, tuberculosis treatment saved 22 million lives between 1995 and 2012. One hundred and one countries, 74 of which are developing, still have increasing HIV incidence. Southern Africa and central Africa, the highest incidence regions, saw sharp declines of 48% and 54%, respectively. Seventy percent (1.6 million cases) of the estimated number of new infections in 2012 occurred in sub-Saharan Africa (Murray et al., 2014; United Nations, 2014).

Although health improvement in sub-Saharan Africa still lags behind many countries and failed to achieve rapid health changes similar to most regions in the world, they made considerable progress in controlling the spread of infectious diseases such as malaria and HIV/AIDS and had a remarkable reduction in child deaths. Globally, there are indicators of a decline in the diseases of poverty, such as communicable diseases and stunting in children under 5 years of age as a result of nutritional problems. Stunting in children under 5 years of age has decreased globally from 40% to 25% over the same period. The percentage of underweight children is estimated to have declined from 25% in 1990 to 15% in 2013 (WHO, 2014). People in wealthier countries live longer and have lower mortality rates; however, conditions such as depression and disabilities have risen. For example, Americans have an increase in life expectancy with more years living with disability including musculoskeletal, mental, and behavioral disorders, such as low back and neck pain, depression, and anxiety. Diseases responsible for the greatest number of years of life lost in the Unites States in 2010 included ischemic heart disease, lung cancer, stroke, chronic obstructive pulmonary disease, and road injury (Institute for Health Metrics and Evaluation: University of Washington, 2013).

The MDGs conclude at the end of 2015, and the proportional contribution of the major cause to the total disease burden is projected to change substantially by 2030, but world leaders have called for a long-term agenda to improve people's lives. Causes related to communicable, maternal, perinatal, and nutritional conditions are projected to account for 20% of total disability-adjusted life years lost in 2030, compared with a little bit lower than 40% in 2004. The noncommunicable disease burden is projected to increase to 66% in 2030 in all income groups. As shown in **Figure 9-1**, the three leading causes of disability-adjusted life years in 2030 are projected

Figure 9-1

Ten Leading Causes of Burden of Disease, World, 2004 and 2030

2004 Disease or injury	As % of total DALYs	Rank		Rank	As % of total DALYs	2030 Disease or injury
Lower respiratory infections	6.2	1		1	6.2	Unipolar depressive disorders
Diarrhoeal diseases	4.8	2		2	5.5	Ischaemic heart disease
Unipolar depressive disorders	4.3	3		3	4.9	Road traffic accidents
Ischaemic heart disease	4.1	4		4	4.3	Cerebrovascular disease
HIV/AIDS	3.8	5		5	3.8	COPD
Cerebrovascular disease	3.1	6		6	3.2	Lower respiratory infections
Prematurity and low birth weight	2.9	7		7	2.9	Hearing loss, adult onset
Birth asphyxia and birth trauma	2.7	8		8	2.7	Refractive errors
Road traffic accidents	2.7	9		9	2.5	HIV/AIDS
Neonatal infections and other[a]	2.7	10		10	2.3	Diabetes mellitus
COPD	2.0	13		11	1.9	Neonatal infections and other[a]
Refractive errors	1.8	14		12	1.9	Prematurity and low birth weight
Hearing loss, adult onset	1.8	15		15	1.9	Birth asphyxia and birth trauma
Diabetes mellitus	1.3	19		18	1.6	Diarrhoeal diseases

Reprinted from World Health Organization. (2012). *The global burden of disease: 2004 update (Figure 27, p. 51).* Retrieved from http://www.who.int/healthinfo/global_burden_disease/GBD_report_2004update_full.pdf

to be unipolar depressive disorders, ischemic heart disease, and road traffic accidents (WHO, 2004). The rise of the importance of noncommunicable diseases in some regions of the developing world has led to calls for goals that cover a broader range of diseases. The United Nations (2015a) responded to this call "by working with governments, civil society and other partners to build on the momentum generated by the MDGs and carry on with an ambitious post-2015 sustainable development agenda that is expected to be adopted by United Nations Member States at the Special Summit on Sustainable Development in September 2015."

Sustainable Development Goals

There are 17 proposed Sustainable Development Goals that follow and expand on the Millennium Development Goals. These goals will be applicable from January 2016 and expected to end in 2030. An example of a sustainable development goal is goal 3, "ensure healthy lives and promote wellbeing for all at all ages" and its aims, which included the three health related MDGs (4, 5, and 6) discussed in this chapter (United Nations, 2014, 2015b). For more in-depth discussion the reader is directed to the following United Nations website: http://www.un.org/sustainabledevelopment/sustainable-development-goals/.

Global Nurse Education and Competencies

It is estimated that 35 million nurses and midwives in the world make up the greatest proportion of the global health workforce; therefore, they need to be properly educated and prepared for global health care. The levels and preparation of initial education for professional nurses varies around the world. Therefore, WHO (2009) established global standards for the initial education of professional nurses and midwives to help countries raise the standards of nursing education and ensure its alignment with worldwide education trends. Many nursing schools in less developed countries have limited access to the latest health and research. To fill that gap, a nursing "Supercourse" website was created that provides a global network of nurses working to improve global health and disease prevention and to expand nursing education worldwide (Shishani et al., 2012). This website followed the inception of, and became part of the "Supercourse: epidemiology, the internet and global health website" at the WHO Collaborating Center University of Pittsburgh, which has a network of over 65,000 scientists in 174 countries and a repository of 5,820 free lectures and courses in 32 languages on global health and disease prevention designed to improve the teaching of prevention (LaPorte, Linkov, & Shubnikov, 2015). The Supercourse website provides epidemiology courses, basic concepts and principles, basic methods, biostatistics, common topics, injuries, cardiovascular disease, cancer, diabetes, legacy lectures, infectious disease, public health, global health, environmental health, family and women's health, children's health, molecular epidemiology, telecommunication, and courses on other topics. The nursing Supercourse website contains lectures driven by global health trends on chronic disease management, clinical issues, family health, health promotion, global health, and nursing education (University of Pittsburgh, 2015).

Another task force that focuses on preparing global health nurses is the Global Alliance for Leadership in Nursing Education and Science (2011), which is composed of nursing associations and councils of deans in the United States, Canada, the United Kingdom, Australia, New Zealand, and South Africa. It serves as the international voice on the contribution of professional nursing education and scholarship to improving global health and health care. It provides strategic expertise in the education and professional development of nurses worldwide to promote global efforts to enhance nursing education and ultimately to prepare nurses who can provide quality health care for the world's populations.

Nursing faculty in the United States, Canada, and Latin America perceived the adapted global health competencies for medical students as essential global health competencies for inclusion in undergraduate nursing curricula despite the fact there is no consensus on global health competencies for medical students (Battat et al., 2010). The 30 identified competencies illustrated in **Table 9-2** are divided into six broad categories: global burden of

Table 9-2

Global Health Competencies and Subscales

I. Global burden of disease

A basic understanding of the global burden of disease is an essential part of a modern nursing education. This knowledge is crucial for participating in discussions of priority setting, health care rationing, and funding for health and health-related research. A nursing graduate should be able to demonstrate the following:

I a. Describe the major causes of morbidity and mortality around the world and how the risk of disease varies with regions

I b. Describe major public health efforts to reduce disparities in global health (such as Millennium Development Goals and Global Fund to Fight AIDS, TB, and malaria)

I c. Discuss priority setting, health care rationing, and funding for health and health-related research

II. Health implications of migration, travel, and displacement

The appropriate management of patients necessitates taking into consideration perspectives and risks posed by international travel or foreign birth. A nursing graduate should be able to:

IIa. Demonstrate an understanding of the health risks posed by international travel or foreign birth

IIb. Recognize when travel or foreign birth places a patient at risk for unusual diseases or unusual presentation of common diseases and make an appropriate assessment or referral

IIc. Describe how cultural context influences perceptions of health and disease

IId. Elicit individual health concerns in a culturally sensitive manner

IIe. Communicate effectively with patients and families using a translator

IIf. Identify world regions and/or travel activities associated with increased risk for life-threatening diseases including HIV/AIDS, malaria, and multidrug-resistant tuberculosis

III. Social and environmental determinants of health

Social, economic, and environmental factors are important determinants of health; furthermore, health is more than simply the absence of disease. Nurses should understand how social, economic, and environmental conditions affect health, both to recognize disease risk factors in their patients and to contribute to improving public health. A nursing graduate should be able to:

IIIa. Describe how social and economic conditions such as poverty, education, and lifestyles affect health and access to health care

IIIb. List major social determinants of health and their impact on differences in life expectancy between and within countries

IIIc. Describe the impact of low income, education, and communication factors on access to and quality of health care

IIId. Describe the relationship between access to clean water, sanitation, food, and air quality on individual and population health

IIIe. Describe the relationship between environmental degradation and human health

IV. Globalization of health and health care

Globalization is profoundly changing disease patterns and the availability of health care workers worldwide. Beside the direct effects of diseases, health care workers and patients moving around the world, global agreements and institutions affect governments' and health care systems' ability to meet populations' health needs. A nursing graduate should be able to:

IVa. Analyze how global trends in health care practice, commerce and culture, multinational agreements, and multinational organizations contribute to the quality and availability of health and health care locally and internationally

IVb. Describe different national models or health systems for provision of health care and their respective effects on health and health care expenditure

IVc. Analyze how travel and trade contribute to the spread of communicable and chronic diseases

IVd. Analyze general trends and influences in the global availability and movement of health care workers

IVe. Describe national and global health care worker availability and shortages

IVf. Describe the most common patterns of health care worker migration and its impact on health care availability in the country that the health care worker leaves and the country to which he or she migrates

V. Health care in low-resource settings

Health care needs and resources markedly differ between high- and low-resource settings, yet much medical training occurs in high-resource settings. To effectively care for patients across a range of settings, a nursing graduate should be able to:

Va. Articulate barriers to health and health care in low-resource settings locally and internationally

Vb. Demonstrate an understanding of cultural and ethical issues in working with disadvantaged populations

Vc. Demonstrate the ability to adapt clinical skills and practice in a resource-constrained setting

Vd. Identify signs and symptoms for common major diseases that facilitate nursing assessment in the absence of advanced testing often unavailable in low-resource settings (cardiovascular disease, cancer, and diabetes)

Ve. Describe the role of syndromic management and clinical algorithms for treatment of common illnesses

Vf. Identify clinical interventions and integrated strategies that have been demonstrated to substantially improve individual and/or population health in low-resource settings (e.g., immunizations, essential drugs, maternal child health programs)

Vg. For students who participate in electives in low-resource settings outside their home situations, a demonstration that they have participated in training to prepare for this elective

VI. Health as a human right and development resource

Human rights impact both individual and population health. Health also is an essential element of economic and social development. To effectively advocate for patients' and communities' health based on an understanding of the relationship between human rights, social and economic development, and health, a nursing graduate should be able to:

VIa. Demonstrate a basic understanding of the relationship between health and human rights

VIb. Demonstrate familiarity with organizations and agreements that address human rights in health care and medical research

VIc. Describe the role of WHO in linking health and human rights, the Universal Declaration of Human Rights, International Ethical Guidelines for Biomedical Research Involving Human Subjects (2002), Declaration of Helsinki (2008)

Reprinted from *Journal of Professional Nursing, 28*(4), Wilson, L., Harper, D., C., Tami-Maury, I., Zarate, R., Salas, S., Farley, J., Ventura, C., Global health competencies for nurses in the Americas, 213-222, Copyright 2012, with permission from Elsevier.

disease; health implications of travel; migration and displacement; social and environmental determinants of health; globalization of health and health care; health care in low resource settings; and health as a human right and development resource (Wilson et al., 2012). However, further research is needed to refine and validate global health competencies to prepare global health nurses.

Global health nurses should be equipped with knowledge and skills to deliver PHC, which are key components in delivering health services to all. Primary health care is still overlooked, and its role is underestimated not only in developing countries but also in parts of the developed countries.

The health system should shift gears from being hospital centered to primary health care (De Maeseneer & Twagirumukiza, 2010; Rao & Pilot, 2014). To better train the health care force, programs should create curricula and training to integrate global health and primary health care training to achieve distinct competencies in both beyond the shared competencies (Truglio et al., 2012).

Primary Health Care in Global Health Nursing

Nurses are among the health care professionals who have always played a pivotal role in the provision of PHC in the global health initiatives by building stable communities and providing services to individuals and populations within their communities, in the United States and worldwide. Nurses are the backbone of health care delivery systems worldwide. According to the Global Nursing Caucus (2015), nurses comprise 50 to 80% of the global health care workforce, providing a variety of care to diverse populations at all levels of the health system in the United States and worldwide. Globalization of the nursing workforce encompasses legal, economic, cultural, social, and educational aspects (Shaffer, 2014). As the world gets smaller and globalization is greater, it is evident that what emerges in the Middle East, Asia, Africa, Europe, and Central Latin America has a contagion effect on the United States, not only on politics, economic, social stability, and education but on health, health policies, health resources, and services.

In response to the need of advancing global health, in November 2013 the Honor Society of Nursing, Sigma Theta Tau International, formed the Global Advisory Panel on the Future of Nursing. In 2015 and 2016, this panel will assemble a series of meetings in the Middle East, Asia/Oceania, the Caribbean, Central Latin America, Africa, Europe, and North America to develop a unified voice and vision for the future of nursing worldwide to advance world health (Klopper & Hill, 2015). Recently, the American Public Health Association updated the 1996 definition of public health nursing to be "the practice of promoting and protecting the health of populations using knowledge from nursing, social, and public health sciences" (American Public Health Association, Public Health Nursing Section, 2013). The second goal of the American Academy of Nursing's (AAN, 2014) strategic plan for 2014 to 2017 is to address the broad range of factors that shape the health of populations so it is consistent with a focus on global health. The president of the AAN declared that this organization would no longer be "American" and would open its doors for fellows from within and outside of the United States. The future vision of the AAN is to achieve global health nursing, which is beyond and broader than international nursing (Mason, 2014).

To best understand nurses' contributions and roles in primary health care, it is wise to view it in the global nursing context. PHC is becoming the essential path for providing health care, and new roles must be developed for PHC nurses (Ross & Mackenzie, 1996). Traditionally, primary health care was seen as care delivered in the community setting, where care may be delivered in a way that is universally accessible to individuals, families, and populations. Today primary health care is seen as care that may be delivered across all health care settings. In order to provide care that is appropriate to the health needs of an increasingly changing global population, professional nurses will have to consider the historic, current, political, social stability, economic, educational, environmental, and cultural factors (multiple determinants of health) as they greatly influence the health and health care services of the population served.

The 2008 WHO report, *Primary Health Care: Now More Than Ever*, focused on the place of PHC in health systems globally and revealed that few changes in PHC have happened since the 1978 WHO Declaration of Alma-Ata. It suggests four PHC reforms that are needed if there is to be continued progress in the attainment of health for all. These include universal coverage reforms that will contribute to health equity and accessibility to all; service delivery reforms that place people at the center of health care, meeting their needs as well as their expectations; reforms in public policy as a means to integrate public health with primary care; and leadership reform that facilitates the engagement of multiple stakeholders in a participatory manner (World Health Organization, 2008). The Office of Nursing and Midwifery at WHO headquarters in Geneva showed its commitment to the global revitalization of PHC by launching a PHC nursing project that collected case studies across the world to illustrate the positive impact of nurses and midwives on health using the PHC approach (Salvage, 2009).

The future of nursing requires establishment of a vision and a voice that addresses key issues including leadership, policy, practice, education, and a qualified workforce. Nurses can contribute significantly to global health and to the goal of health for all at the local, national, and international levels through PHC initiatives, helping to address the challenges associated with the global nursing shortage and international nurse migration, promoting global health equity through leadership and involvement in health policy development, and participating in international exchanges and collaborations (Anderson & McFarlane, 2015).

Examples of Primary Health Care Practice Globally

It is important to remember that building a health care system that embraces the essential elements of primary health care is country specific and very much depends on the history and varied experiences of that country, including the acknowledgment of health for all, public health infrastructure, political policies, cultural awareness, economic feasibility, educational foundations, and the variety of resources necessary to build and sustain a comprehensive health care system. No one health care system will encapsulate each and every essential element of primary health care. What is important for this discussion is the recognition that each country and each health care system that is evolving is doing so within the country's capacity and based on the needs of the people. Key to this is the belief that health is an essential human right. The case exemplars that follow provide examples of growing and evolving primary health care practices globally. As you read, reflect on each of the cases and its relationship with the Declaration of Alma-Ata. Take time to address the following questions once you have considered the case:

1. What is it about this case exemplar that reflects the principles of primary health care?
2. In what way(s) can the providers and participants, within the case exemplar, develop and expand upon the principles of primary health care practices?
3. What leadership roles do nurses need to play in these initiatives?

Case Study 1: Primary Health Care Mission to Haiti

In 2014, an interdisciplinary health care team, comprised of nurses, physicians, a pharmacist, and a social worker from Pusan National University Yangsan Hospital, South Korea, and 12 faculty, staff, and students from the School of Nursing at the George Washington University, United States, partnered to provide health services and health promotion education for almost 3,000 medically underserved people in the Caracol and neighboring Cap Haitian area of Haiti. The health services included a pediatric clinic treating parasitic and skin infections, maternal-child health and development, adult general medicine clinic, and triage that focused on screening for hypertension and diabetes. Registered nurses, nurse practitioners, nursing students, and physicians worked together in the shared goal to improve the health of the Haitian people and their community through integrated health services and health education programs. Drawing on prioritized health needs and challenges affecting Haiti and its people, the health promotion activities related to specific health education topics including recognizing and lowering high blood pressure, nutrition to support healthy choices, pediatric oral rehydration, hand sanitation, food safety, preventing sexually transmitted infections (STIs), and gender violence. Educational materials such as posters, videos, and oral presentations were designed and presented by student nurses, translated and delivered in the native language, Creole. This annual short-term health care mission provides primary health care services to those whose health care needs frequently go unmet. The PHC clinic is supported by university primary partners, private and public donations, and the government of Haiti. Primary health care clinics in rural Haiti provide a unique opportunity for interdisciplinary collaboration between two universities, a teaching hospital, local and national agencies, and government and nongovernment organizations to provide primary health care services based on immediate, prevailing, and emerging health problems in one of the poorest countries in the Western Hemisphere (Lang, Whitlow, Johnson, & Pulcini, 2015).

Case Study 2: Primary Health Care Mental Health Clinic in the United States

The integration of primary health care in a mental health center project in the United States involved collaboration between a community behavioral health center, a local hospital, and a university school of nursing to design primary health care services for patients with serious mental illness. The Primary Health Care Clinic, located within the community mental health center, provided screening for acute illness, management of chronic disease, and "well person" physical exams, mental health services, and educational programs aimed at promoting health and preventing disease. The goal of the clinic was to prevent/reduce potential complications from common health problems by making health services more accessible, thereby reducing long waits and delays in seeking treatment. Health services were provided by a nurse practitioner, faculty member who coordinated care with mental health providers, case managers, and staff who supported integration of high-quality, individualized primary health care services in a supportive environment (Stevens & Sidlinger, 2015).

Case Study 3: Primary Health Care Nurse-Led Mobile Chemotherapy Clinic in the United Kingdom

A nurse-led mobile chemotherapy clinic, the first of its kind in the United Kingdom, provided chemotherapy services normally offered in the acute care setting to cancer patients living in rural communities. The initiative, supported by the United Kingdom Department of Health (DH), was to implement a more efficient way to provide chemotherapy care closer to home as well as support services to cancer patients who were traveling long distances to receive chemotherapy care. The nurse-led mobile clinic was successful in expanding services to rural communities in the United Kingdom. Patients reported significant savings in time spent traveling, expenditure on fuel, and companion costs. In addition, they were pleased with the available car parking. Patient's stress and boredom were lowered by shorter wait times to receive the treatment and the more informal procedures in the mobile clinic. The environment in the mobile clinic was friendly, so patients were able to talk more to nurses and other patients. This mobile chemotherapy unit is an innovative way to deliver tertiary care within a primary health care perspective. In addition, this method supports patients having access to their treatment within the community and further facilitates providers have access to their patients (Mitchell, 2013).

Case Study 4: Nurse-Led Open Access Iron Deficiency Anemia Primary Health Care Clinic in the United Kingdom

In the United Kingdom, the current wait time between referral and endoscopic diagnosis of gastrointestinal (GI) cancer is approximately 11 weeks. This waiting time is unacceptable for critical early diagnosis and timely treatment interventions. A nurse-led clinic was created to "fast track" patients presenting with signs or symptoms of gastrointestinal cancer for prompt referral for endoscopic diagnosis. Patients were seen by a clinical nurse specialist who evaluated signs and symptoms of gastrointestinal cancer. Over a 15-month period, 100% of the patients referred by the clinical nurse specialist received an endoscopic examination, and 19 patients were found to have gastrointestinal cancer. This nurse-led primary care clinic was highly successful in achieving the goals of improving referral to diagnosis, and the clinical nurse specialist was capable of assessing these patients and planning appropriate investigations (Davis, Bowman, & Shepherd, 2004). In addition, this nurse-led clinic was "open access," thus enhancing accessibility.

Case Study 5: Primary Health Care Nurses Training in South Africa

Another example of primary health care in action is described by Ravhura, Gumede, and Dipholo (2014). The study examined the relationship between primary health care learning programs and health care service delivery and how they benefited the local community. The researchers wanted to determine the difference between the quality of services provided in health care facilities using primary health care–trained nurses and those using nurses without primary health care training. A functional difference was found in the scope of practice between nurses trained and those not trained in primary health care. As a result of these positive findings, the authors "strongly recommended that all professional nurses in primary health care facilities should be trained in the learning programs in order to strengthen the primary health care system" (Ravhura et al., 2014, p. 207). Several insights were gained from this research: (1) challenges and trajectory of successful interprofessional team building with different organizational goals and cultural perspectives; (2) the organization of services to serve large numbers of patients including what worked well and challenges encountered in organizing a health care service with limited resources; and (3) patient demographic characteristics, range of symptoms mentioned, and unique health promotion/disease prevention efforts. Lessons learned from this study will guide future nursing curriculum in PHC nursing.

Case Study 6: Nurses Nutritional Advice to Pregnant Women in Saudi Arabia

This joint research program between British and Saudi Arabian universities provided nutritional advice to pregnant women attending a primary health care center in Saudi Arabia. Information was provided using culturally sensitive approaches appropriate to Islamic teaching and Saudi culture, using the Qur'an as the framework of primary health care. This culturally appropriate program is congruent with the cultural beliefs, life ways, and customs of the country and its people, which is crucial in addressing World Health Organization and International Council of Nursing objectives. Contextualizing benefits to the community is a key component in PHC nursing whether at home or in another country. Female nurses have a low status in Saudi Arabia, and the primarily male-dominated medical system presented a challenge to the female interviewer. However, this challenge was overcome through understanding the cultural patterns and views and beliefs about health and wellness. The authors found that the Western practice of nursing—which is primarily focused on the individual, autonomy, and promotes self-care—is less applicable in Saudi Arabia and unlikely to be applicable in countries with a similar social structure (Littlewood & Yousuf, 2000).

Summary

Nurses no longer have to travel to the most remote places on earth to practice global nursing; many opportunities exist to work with individuals and communities from diverse cultural, ethnic, and international backgrounds in their own country. The world is rapidly changing, and so is health and health care. It is crucial that today's nurses understand the current, prevailing, and emerging health problems and health care challenges not only in their own country but around the world. Collaborative work globally should be fostered to prepare global nurses with the knowledge, competencies, and skills for the 21st century so they can deliver primary health care efficiently to save and improve people's lives.

Chapter Activities

1. Describe the relevance of one or two of the Millennium Development Goals (MDG) to your practice population. How might you promote that goal within your own practice setting?

2. Compare primary health care–focused delivery systems in a developed country with a health care delivery system without this focus in a developing country. Then list the specific inputs necessary to integrate primary health care nursing to promote health care delivery.

3. Using the Declaration of the Alma-Alta as a guide, review how developed and developing countries address the concept of primary health care and health as a human right for all. What can international health care systems learn from each other in promoting the health of the country and its people? What are the policy implications of your findings?

4. Conduct an Internet search of global health websites to identify immediate, prevailing, and emerging global health issues. For example, look at the World Health Organization (WHO), Pan American Health Organization (PAHO), Centers for Disease Control and Prevention (CDC), United States Agency for International Development (USAID), the United Nations Children's Fund (UNICEF), and the World Bank.

5. Discuss current approaches utilized by various countries to address health problems and issues facing the country and its people, and consider primary health care approaches to facilitate improvements and change. For example, how might primary health care nurses identify and target high-risk populations, initiate hand sanitation and food safety education programs, and evaluate its effects in reducing morbidity and mortality in the recent cholera outbreak in Haiti?

6. In a small group, discuss and propose specific interventions based on prioritized health needs of a target population to address global health concerns. Consider disparities in health care access, services, and resources in a selected underdeveloped country.

7. How might you use the information in this chapter to reflect on how you use global nursing to promote primary health care in your own practice?

References

American Academy of Nursing. (2014). *Strategic goals 2014–2017*. Retrieved from http://www.aannet.org/strategic-plan-2014-2017

American Public Health Association, Public Health Nursing Section. (2013). *The definition and practice of public health nursing*. Retrieved from http://www.apha .org/~/media/files/pdf/membergroups/nursingdefinition.ashx

Anderson, E. T., & McFarlane, J. M. (2015). *Community as partner: Theory and practice in nursing*. Philadelphia, PA: Wolters Kluwer Health.

Battat, R., Seidman, G., Chadi, N., Chanda, M. Y., Nehme, J., Hulme, J.,... Brewer, T. F. (2010). Global health competencies and approaches in medical education: A literature review. *BMC Medical Education, 10*, 94–94. doi:10.1186/1472-6920-10-94

Brown, T. M., Cueto, M., & Fee, E. (2006). The world health organization and the transition from "international" to "global" public health. *American Journal of Public Health, 96*(1), 62–72. Retrieved from http://search.ebscohost.com/login .aspx?direct=true&db=s3h&AN=19347222&site=ehost-live

Campbell, R. M., Pleic, M., & Connolly, H. (2012). The importance of a common global health definition: How Canada's definition influences its strategic direction in global health. *Journal of Global Health, 2*(1), 010301–010301. doi:10.7189/jogh.02.010301

Centers for Disease Control and Prevention. (2014). *CDC global health strategy 2012–2015*. Retrieved from http://www.cdc.gov/globalhealth/strategy/pdf/CDC -GlobalHealthStrategy.pdf

Davis, A., Bowman, D., & Shepherd, H. A. (2004). Patients referred from primary care with iron-deficiency anaemia: Analysis of a nurse-led service. An improvement for both doctor and patient? *Quality in Primary Care, 12*(2), 129–135. Retrieved from http://search.ebscohost.com/login.aspx?direct=true &db=rzh&AN=2005029684&site=ehost-live

De Maeseneer, J., & Twagirumukiza, M. (2010). The contribution of primary health care to global health. *The British Journal of General Practice: The Journal of the Royal College of General Practitioners, 60*(581), 875–876. doi:10.3399/bjgp10X543998

Global Nursing Caucus. (2015). *Engaging nurses to advance global health*. Retrieved from http://www.globalnursingcaucus.org/resources/advocacy/

Institute for Health Metrics and Evaluation. (2015a). *History*. Retrieved from http:// www.healthdata.org/about/history

Institute for Health Metrics and Evaluation. (2015b). *About GBD*. Retrieved from http://www.healthdata.org/gbd/about

Institute for Health Metrics and Evaluation: University of Washington. (2013). *The state of US health: Innovations, insights, and recommendations from the global burden of disease study*. Retrieved from http://www.healthdata.org/sites /default/files/files/policy_report/2013/USHealth/IHME_GBD_USHealth _FullReport.pdf

Kassebaum, N. J., Bertozzi-Villa, A., Coggeshall, M. S., Shackelford, K. A., Steiner, C., Heuton, K. R.,... Lozano, R. (2014). Global, regional, and national levels and causes of maternal mortality during 1990–2013: A systematic analysis for the global burden of disease study 2013. *Lancet (North American Edition), 384*(9947), 980–1004. Retrieved from http://search.ebscohost.com/login.aspx

?direct=true&db=bxh&AN=BACD201400526892&site=ehost-live; http://www
.thelancet.com/

Khubchandani, J. (2012). Going global: Building a foundation for global health promotion research to practice. *Health Promotion Practice, 13*(3), 293–297.

Klopper, H. C., & Hill, M. (2015). Global advisory panel on the future of nursing (GAPFON) and global health. *Journal of Nursing Scholarship, 47*(1), 3–4. doi:10.1111/jnu.12118

Koplan, J. P., Bond, T. C., Merson, M. H., Reddy, K. S., Rodriguez, M. H., Sewankambo, N. K., & Wasserheit, J. N. (2009). Towards a common definition of global health. *The Lancet, 373*(9679), 1993–1995. Retrieved from http://search.proquest .com.proxygw.wrlc.org/docview/199047004?accountid=11243

Lang, C., Whitlow, M., Johnson, J., & Pulcini, J. (2015). *Primary health care mission to Haiti.* Unpublished manuscript.

LaPorte, R., Linkov, F., & Shubnikov, F. (2015). *Supercourse epidemiology, the Internet and global health.* Retrieved from http://www.pitt.edu/~super1/#

Littlewood, J., & Yousuf, S. (2000). Primary health care in Saudi Arabia: Applying global aspects of health for all, locally. *Journal of Advanced Nursing, 32*(3), 675–681. doi:10.1046/j.1365-2648.2000.01527.x

Mason, D. J. (2014). Think globally, act locally. *Nursing Outlook, 62*(1), 5–6. doi:10.1016/j.outlook.2013.11.005

Mitchell, T. (2013). Patients' experiences of receiving chemotherapy in outpatient clinic and/or onboard a unique nurse-led mobile chemotherapy unit: A qualitative study. *European Journal of Cancer Care, 22*(4), 430–439. Retrieved from http://search.ebscohost.com/login.aspx?direct=true&db=psyh&AN=2013 -21848-004&site=ehost-live

Murray, C. J. L., Ortblad, K. F., Guinovart, C., Lim, S. S., Wolock, T. M., Roberts, D. A.,... Vos, T. (2014). Global, regional, and national incidence and mortality for HIV, tuberculosis, and malaria during 1990–2013: A systematic analysis for the global burden of disease study 2013. *Lancet (North American Edition), 384*(9947), 1005–1070. Retrieved from http://search.ebscohost.com/login.asp x?direct=true&db=bxh&AN=BACD201400526893&site=ehost-live; http://www .thelancet.com/

Rao, M., & Pilot, E. (2014). The missing link—The role of primary care in global health. *Global Health Action, 7,* 1–6. doi:10.3402/gha.v7.23693

Ravhura, J. H., Gumede, N., & Dipholo, K. (2014). The effect of primary health care learning program in health care service delivery: Case study of Ehlanzeni health district in Mpumalanga province. *Journal of Educational and Social Research, 4*(6), 207–220.

Ross, F., & Mackenzie, A. (1996). *Nursing in primary health care: Policy and practice.* London and New York: Routledge.

Salvage, J. (2009). Global revitalisation of primary health care. *Primary Health Care, 19*(1), 16–17. Retrieved from http://search.ebscohost.com/login.aspx?direct =true&db=rzh&AN=2010201938&site=ehost-live

Shaffer, F. A. (2014). Ensuring a global workforce: A challenge and opportunity. *Nursing Outlook, 62*(1), 1–4. doi:10.1016/j.outlook.2013.08.001

Shishani, K., Allen, C., Shubnikov, E., Salman, K., Laporte, R. E., & Linkov, F. (2012). Nurse educators establishing new venues in global nursing education. *Journal of Professional Nursing, 28*(2), 132–134. doi:10.1016/j.profnurs.2011.11.008

Stevens, C., & Sidlinger, L. (2015). Integration of primary care into a mental health center: Lessons learned from year one implementation. *Kansas Nurse, 90*(1), 12–15. Retrieved from http://search.ebscohost.com/login.aspx?direct=true&db=rzh&AN=2012857367&site=ehost-live

Truglio, J., Graziano, M., Vedanthan, R., Hahn, S., Rios, C., Hendel-Paterson, B., & Ripp, J. (2012). Global health and primary care: Increasing burden of chronic diseases and need for integrated training. *Mount Sinai Journal of Medicine, 79*(4), 464–474. doi:10.1002/msj.21327

United Nations. (2014). *The millennium development goals report 2014.* Retrieved from http://www.un.org/millenniumgoals/2014%20MDG%20report/MDG%202014%20English%20web.pdf

United Nations. (2015a). *Millennium development goals and beyond 2015.* Retrieved from http://www.un.org/millenniumgoals/beyond2015-overview.shtml

United Nations. (2015b). *Open working group on sustainable development goals.* Retrieved from https://sustainabledevelopment.un.org/owg.html

University of Pittsburgh. (2015). *Nursing supercourse.* Retrieved from http://www.pitt.edu/~super1/collections/collection44.htm

Wang, H., Liddell, C. A., Coates, M. M., Mooney, M. D., Levitz, C. E., Schumacher, A. E.,… Liu, S. (2014). Global, regional, and national levels of neonatal, infant, and under-5 mortality during 1990–2013: A systematic analysis for the global burden of disease study 2013. *Lancet, 384*(9947), 957–979. Retrieved from http://search.ebscohost.com/login.aspx?direct=true&db=her&AN=98277839&site=ehost-live

Wilson, L., Harper, D. C., Tami-Maury, I., Zarate, R., Salas, S., Farley, J.,… Ventura, C. (2012). Global health competencies for nurses in the Americas. *Journal of Professional Nursing, 28*(4), 213–222. doi:10.1016/j.profnurs.2011.11.021

World Health Organization. (2004). *The global burden of disease: 2004 update.* Retrieved from http://www.who.int/healthinfo/global_burden_disease/GBD_report_2004update_full.pdf

World Health Organization. (2008). *The world health report 2008—Primary health care: Now more than ever.* Retrieved from http://www.who.int/whr/2008/whr08_en.pdf

World Health Organization. (2009). *Global standards for the initial education of professional nurses and midwives.* Retrieved from http://www.who.int/hrh/nursing_midwifery/hrh_global_standards_education.pdf

World Health Organization. (2014). *MDG 1: Eradicate extreme poverty and hunger.* Retrieved from http://www.who.int/topics/millennium_development_goals/hunger/en/

World Health Organization. (2015a). *Alert, response, and capacity building under the international health regulations (IHR).* Retrieved from http://www.who.int/ihr/publications/9789241596664/en/

World Health Organization. (2015b). *Public health: Trade, foreign policy, diplomacy and health.* Retrieved from http://www.who.int/trade/glossary/story076/en/

Chapter 10

Culturally Sensitive Primary Health Care Interventions: Three Exemplars

Arlene W. Keeling, Brigid Lusk, and Pamela K. Kulbok

Chapter Objectives

By the end of this chapter, you will be able to:

1. Compare historical precedents and implications of culturally sensitive primary health care based on two case exemplars: the Navajo, 1920–1950; and post-mastectomy patients, 1950–1960.

2. Examine community participation as a primary health care strategy to enhance cultural sensitivity and for the development of culturally congruent strategies in contemporary rural America.

Since the inception of professional nursing in 1873 with the opening of the first nurse training schools in the United States, nurses have been involved in developing and implementing primary health care initiatives. Nurses' role in promoting health expanded with the initiation of visiting nurses' associations in the late 19th century and the inception of the term and practice of *public health nursing* led by nurse leader Lillian Wald. Early on, visiting and public health nurses understood the importance of providing culturally congruent care. This chapter explores three case studies, two historical and one contemporary, in which nurses developed interventions and health teaching that were sensitive to the culture of those receiving care. Highlighting nurses working in the Indian Health Service and those caring for cancer patients post-mastectomy in the mid-20th century, the chapter traces the importance of cultural competence in a primary health care (PHC) practice. The chapter concludes with a more recent example of nurses working with rural adolescent teens, which demonstrates that culturally competent care is still important today.

Nurses on the Navajo Reservation, 1920s–1950

In the mid-1920s, the U.S. Secretary of the Interior commissioned Lewis Meriam, a medical specialist employed by the Department of the Interior, to conduct a survey of the health services provided to the American Indians. The results, published in 1928 in the *Meriam Report,* were graphic in detail, describing extreme poverty, poor health and nutrition, and a lack of sanitation among the Indians. In addition, the report documented inadequate salaries for physicians and nurses, inadequate medical facilities, a dearth of public health nurses, and minimal efforts toward preventive medicine. It also confirmed the fact that the two "great health problems" were tuberculosis and trachoma (Meriam, 1928, p. 201).

Based on the survey results, the American Red Cross recommended "the immediate establishment of an organized public health nursing service as part of the Indian health program" (Meriam, 1928, p. 20) and assigned three trained Red Cross nurses as visiting nurses to Navajo reservations in a trial program. Between 1924 and 1934, the number of field nurses employed by the government grew from 3 to 98. The nurses who applied to the Indian Health Service (IHS) were, for the most part, White and middle class, reflecting the typical nurse of the era. Many were seeking adventure and travel. They found it. Far from home and living on the Navajo reservation, the young nurses were challenged by the new culture. The chronic physician shortage, the vast distances between the patients' homes (hogans) on the reservation, and extreme weather conditions often resulted in nurses working alone or accompanied only by their Navajo drivers. Field nurse Mary Eppich lamented the fact in one of her monthly reports, writing: "Have had several sick patients at the hogans and have wanted Dr. Stephenson to see them, but he has not made any clinics this month" (Eppich, 1935, p. 1). When their Indian drivers were also unavailable, the nurses made home visits by themselves (Abel, 1996).

Practicing under these conditions, the IHS nurses did whatever they had to do to care for the Navajo people, negotiating weather, travel, professional boundaries, and the Navajo culture to do so. In April 1933, Elizabeth Forster saw 397 patients in her dispensary and made 65 Hogan visits (Forster, 1933). In May 1935, Nena Seymour made home visits to "76 different Hogans," treating "sore throats, ear infections, cuts, impetigo and other commonly occurring diseases"(Seymour, 1935, p. 2).

One of the challenges for the nurses was that of negotiating their role between the White American contract doctors and the Navajo medicine men. The field nurses, trained in traditional nursing programs throughout the United States, accepted without question the validity and efficacy of scientific American medicine (Abel & Reifel, 1999). Now, working on the reservation, they began to realize the importance of understanding the Navajo culture and its core value: maintaining balance and order. For the nurses, accepting the Navajo values would be important to establishing a sense of trust. Traditional healing ceremonies were at the core of Navajo health beliefs and had to be incorporated into the treatment the nurses recommended if the nurses' recommendations were to be taken seriously. Delores Young, RN, commented on that fact: "With the younger Indians who were undecided as to which medicine was the best, it was important to let them have both if they wanted it" (Young, n.d., p. 1). Another nurse, Mary Zillatas (n.d.), noted that she "tried to show the Indians that both cultures could be used to their advantage." Both of these nurses worked according to recommendations in the *Meriam Report*: "The position taken . . . is that the work with and for the Indians must give consideration to the desires of the individual Indians" (Meriam, 1928, p. 88).

Of note, many Navajo were accepting of Western medicines, particularly for diseases they considered to be brought to their reservation by White men. One of the most troublesome diseases that plagued the Navajo was trachoma, a highly contagious disease that ran rampant on the reservation. Aggravated by the hot desert climate as well as dust and wind, trachoma caused granular bumps on the inside of a patient's eyelids. When these scratched the cornea, the patient experienced excruciating pain. Left untreated, the disease eventually resulted in blindness. The field nurses held specialty clinics to address the problem, traveling to isolated areas of the reservation to set up trachoma clinics. Reporting on her work, Nina Seymour (1935) noted: "My Mexican Springs dispensary is at last painted and I set up clinics. Routine trachoma treatments have been started. I have set aside 7:30-9:00 a.m. for trachoma treatments" (p. 2). Realizing that the White man's medicine not only relieved their pain and itching, but also helped them preserve their eyesight, the ever-practical Navajo bypassed their traditional cures for the disease, willingly attending these specialty clinics for treatment.

Thus, rather than force "White man's medicine" on the Navajo, the field nurses tried to establish a sense of trust with the Navajo community so that they then could introduce Anglo-American medicine, culture, health practices, and health beliefs. The first step in this process was for the nurse to accept the Navajo culture. The Navajo believed that "the system of life is one inter-connected whole" and that "the whole human creature—body, mind and spirit" should be treated (Alvord & Van Pelt, 1999, p. 40). This holistic perspective resonated with nurses. Nonetheless, there were some significant aspects of Navajo culture that were foreign to the increasingly scientific American nursing practices in the first half of the 20th century. A major component of the Navajo medicine men's treatment involved "Sings" or "Chantways"—ceremonial chants sung over the patient (Bahti, 2000). One of these, called "Beauty Way," was meant to restore balance to the patient and was based on the Navajo belief that an imbalance in any area of a person's life could cause illness. Other ceremonial Chantways included Lifeway, Blessingway, Enemyway, the Night Chant, the Mountain Way, and Shooting Way. Different chants were meant to cure different illnesses. A "Shooting Way" ceremony might be used to cure an illness thought to have been caused by a snake, lightening, or an arrow; a Lifeway ceremony was used to cure an illness caused by an accident, and so on (Alvord & Van Pelt, 1999, p. 186).

In an attempt to show respect for the Navajo culture, some nurses did not interfere with the "sings" even though they may have wanted to impose their own recommendations. Dorothy Williams, RN, recounted one visit to a hogan to see a child with a broken leg, noting:

> I advised hospital for child [*sic*] but the family said they had already sent for the medicine man and would send the child to hospital in a few days if he failed to cure the leg. I visited the hogan a few days later and found they were still having a "Sing." (Williams, 1935, p. 2)

While she may have been discouraged by the parents' refusal to send the child to the hospital immediately, Williams did not press the issue, and instead, waited for the medicine men to decide to do something different. Sometimes they did, turning to White man's medicine as a last resort. Others accepted the nurses' therapy as an adjunct treatment to their chants. As a result, the nurses often negotiated a treatment regimen somewhere between that recommended by the contract doctor and that prescribed by the Hitachi (Frisbie, 1987). Mary Eppich (1935) described one such case: "[a baby] age 1 year, also has symptoms of Catarrhal Fever. A Sing is being held over him. My treatment was Castor Oil and Aspirin Grains 1 every four hours, plenty of water and not much food" (p. 2). Clearly, Eppich recognized the legitimate power of the medicine men within the community and the importance of working *with* them rather than undermining their authority. Other nurses did the same. Gladys Solveson (1936) described the results of that collaboration, noting:

It has been gratifying to realize that we have gained the confidence of several of the better known medicine men. We have been called frequently this month by the medicine men, both to their own homes as well as to "sings," to consult regarding their patients. Frequently the medicine man has advised the family to consider hospital care when we recommended it. We have brought in a good number of patients who had never seen the inside of a hospital before. (p. 2)

The medicine men's cooperation was essential to any consideration of hospitalization, and sometimes that cooperation was forthcoming. Like their patients, many of the medicine men believed that White man's medicine was better in curing what they referred to as "White men's diseases"—whooping cough, smallpox, measles, tuberculosis, and so forth (Trennert, 1998, p. 33). As one nurse reported:

Recently we advised an influential medicine man to hospitalize his 13 year old boy. The boy had been sick six days and had a temperature of 104 degrees. A "sing" was in progress and several medicine men were present. After a discussion of about an hour and a half, the medicine men decided to send the patient to the hospital. (Solveson, 1936, pp. 1-2)

In her final report to the National Association of Indian Affairs in 1933, Elizabeth Forster (1933), RN, wrote: "I believe that the Red Rock Navajos were beginning to accept me as a friend.... It was gratifying to have them voluntarily invite me to their ceremonies and sand paintings and to find the Medicine Men very willing to cooperate on increasingly frequent occasions" (p. 2). Gaining the trust of these respected community leaders was essential if the nurses were to be effective.

Reflections

The historical papers, written reports, and work of the public health nurses reflect primary health care principles. For example, gathering population-based data via survey design showed the vulnerability of the population of Navajo American Indians because of poverty, poor health, lack of nutrition, and sanitation—all determinants of health. Major health issues that included a high incidence of tuberculosis and trachoma further challenged the health of this population. Compounding the situation was the added realization that this population had limited access to care from any providers, further increasing their vulnerability. These early nurses responded to a call to go to the Navajo people and "reach" them where they live in their home communities where care would be provided. It was clear to these nurses that just by going to the people did not mean that they were going to "reach" the Navajo people, and that working with this population was going to take building trust and respect, which required negotiation so that population-based issues could be addressed. Furthermore, it was clear to these nurses that there was a need, on their part, to fully understand the Navajo way; their ideas, values, and belief systems and relinquish any sense of cultural authority that they may harbor. As these nurses worked in these communities, their ability to "see" all perspectives so that aspects of both cultures could be accepted and blended was crucial as they worked "with" the Navajo to develop plans to address the critical issues. Finally, these nurses identified that working with medicine men was an important strategy for them because these individuals were "key" people for the Navajo people.

Nurses Caring for Women Following Radical Mastectomy, 1950–1960

"My husband got sick to his stomach when he saw my wound" mourned a woman in 1955 following her radical mastectomy (Dericks, 1954–1955, n.p.). Such extensive surgery was the optimal standard of care offered to women with breast cancer in the 1950s; as late as 1968, nearly 70% of women with breast cancer underwent a radical mastectomy (Lerner, 2001, p. 4). Initially devised by American surgeons Willy Meyer and William Halsted around the turn of the 20th century, the radical mastectomy was an attempt to remove all cancerous cells (Haagensen, 1950). The breast, lymph nodes, and both pectoral muscles of the chest wall were removed in a "one-step" excision, with skin grafts applied to cover the cavernous wound. The deformities created by such surgeries were horrible. Women were left disfigured, with a breast and muscles on one side and breast, muscle, nodes, and possibly even rib evisceration on the other. In many women, the arm on the affected side became permanently swollen with lymph. In 1937, British surgeon Geoffrey Keynes called the radical mastectomy "a truly hideous mutilation" (Lerner, 2001, p. 53). It is not surprising that post-mastectomy depression related to the disease and its treatment was common (Renneker & Cutler, 1952).

Cancer in the 1950s, as now, was a particularly feared diagnosis. The word itself carried a stigma, and the threat of death was very real (Patterson, 1991). In 1950, cancer killed more women between 40 and 60 years of age than any other disease, and the breast was the most common site for cancer to strike (Haagensen, 1950). In this context, women's concerns about the potential disfigurement of a radical mastectomy were "a matter of very little importance as compared with the life of the patient" (Halsted, 1894–1895, p. 311). In the 1950s, surgeons still considered a woman's breast as redundant and expendable (Lerner, 2001, p. 89). Thus, these women—in hospital and at home, young and old, of every race and ethnicity—were linked through their culture of fear, cancer phobia, and radical mastectomy.

Let us briefly look at the culture of women in 1950s America. A woman's role was to marry and raise a family, and according to the mores of the time, she needed to "attract and keep" a man primarily through her looks (Smith, 1950, p. 338), which included generously endowed breasts—think of Marilyn Monroe or Jane Russell. As Terese Lasser (1953) opened in *Reach for Recovery*, "Let us begin with the problem which is always a primary concern to all women—their appearance" (p. 8). For a woman with breast cancer, her appearance and her role as a woman, in marriage, motherhood, and female sexuality, was threatened by a mastectomy (Alexander, 1957; Dericks, 1951–1958; Renneker & Cutler, 1952), The images in **Figure 10-1** are taken from educational pamphlets for post-mastectomy patients: Helen Radler's 1954, *A Handbook for Your Recovery*, and Teresa Lasser's 1953, *Reach for Recovery*. They illustrate, through showing the well-adjusted, recovered patient on the arm of "her man," the envisioned height of 1950s female fulfillment.

In 1950s, America gender imbalance was much more pronounced than it is today. Men typically held positions of leadership and power; surgeons, at the height of their professional authority, were invariably male and their patients with breast cancer, along with their nurses, were invariably female.

Figure 10-1

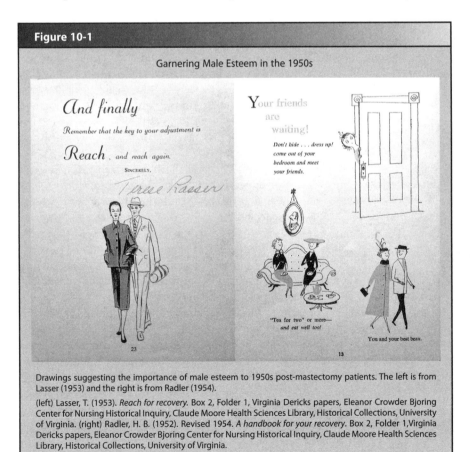

Garnering Male Esteem in the 1950s

Drawings suggesting the importance of male esteem to 1950s post-mastectomy patients. The left is from Lasser (1953) and the right is from Radler (1954).

(left) Lasser, T. (1953). *Reach for recovery*. Box 2, Folder 1, Virginia Dericks papers, Eleanor Crowder Bjoring Center for Nursing Historical Inquiry, Claude Moore Health Sciences Library, Historical Collections, University of Virginia. (right) Radler, H. B. (1952). Revised 1954. *A handbook for your recovery*. Box 2, Folder 1,Virginia Dericks papers, Eleanor Crowder Bjoring Center for Nursing Historical Inquiry, Claude Moore Health Sciences Library, Historical Collections, University of Virginia.

It is illustrative to note here that when First Lady Betty Ford, in the 1970s, underwent a radical mastectomy, she—like most women in her situation—authorized her husband to consent to her radical surgery while she lay anesthetized (Lerner, 2001, p. 175).

Adding to the woman's anxiety and dependence was her ignorance of the cancer diagnosis. In a review of post-mastectomy patients from 1954 to 1962, many examples were found of patients who were not told their diagnosis but had fears they couldn't voice, such as one woman who "does not definitely know the diagnosis is cancer but suspects it" (Dericks, 1951–1967, n.p.). One surgeon/nurse team wrote, "Such vital knowledge had better be shared only with those responsible for the patient's welfare" (Sugarbaker & Wilfley, 1950, p. 338).

Case Study: Nursing Care of Post-Mastectomy Patients, 1950–1960

Nurse Genevieve Waples Smith underwent a radical mastectomy sometime shortly before 1950. "After a rather stormy recovery," she wrote, I "found that my arm on the affected side was very painful and I could lift it only waist high. I was impressed by the lack of any planned care, knowing that I had been as guilty as others in this respect.... The psychological problem, however, is probably the major one. I have heard doctors tell medical and nursing students what a mutilating operation a radical mastectomy is—but with never a suggestion as to how they might make it seem less traumatic to the patient" (Smith, 1950, p. 336).

Some nurses attempted to decrease the trauma. One was Virginia Dericks, an instructor and supervisor in Surgical Nursing at Cornell University—New York Hospital from 1943 to 1962. She worried that the population of radical mastectomy patients was not getting, in her words, "the right kind of care" (personal communication, 2004). In 1954, Dericks formed a committee to strategize how to promote physical and psychological health among these women. The Committee to Improve Nursing Care of Mastectomy Patients included nurses from out-patient and in-patient areas, visiting nurses, private duty nurses, and nursing faculty (personal communication, 2004). The aims were "to improve the nursing care of patients undergoing radical mastectomy, with especial reference to psychological adjustment, post-operative exercises, prosthesis, and clothing" (Dericks, 1954–1958, n.p.). Because this was a nursing problem, Dericks invited only nurses to serve on her committee (personal communication, 2004). The committee members investigated post-mastectomy nursing care through interviewing patients and experienced nurses from hospitals, clinics, and doctors' offices. They also reviewed the files of post-mastectomy patients covering the previous 5 years, 1949 to 1954 (Dericks, 1954–1958).

Terese Lasser (1953), a post-mastectomy patient herself, reminded women that the surgeon was a "busy man, and, being a man he cannot always foresee the many questions which beset a woman." Dericks's patients were routinely scheduled to meet with knowledgeable nurses who took time to answer their intimate questions. The positive effect of these meetings included "one patient [who] felt she was 'too old' to wear a false appliance" but after her meeting she decided to buy one. "On her next clinic visit, there was noticed a decided improvement in her morale, her clothes fit more stylishly, and she had a brighter outlook" (Dericks, 1954–1955, n.p.).

Dericks observed that mastectomy patients experienced great stress at predictable times, including the first time the dressing was changed, when patients looked at their wound for the first time, and when they dressed to go home. She wanted a nurse present with patients to support them at these critical moments (Dericks, 1954–1966). Dericks further advised that patients who were being discharged should be referred to the visiting nurse service for psychological support at home (Dericks, 1954–1955). Much of the data Dericks and her committee gathered came from visiting nurses, and they had seen the support these nurses could offer. The committee also noted that it was helpful for the patient's (male) doctor to talk to her husband "because the attitude of a married woman with a breast removed seems so dependent on her husband's acceptance and understanding of her" (Dericks, 1954–1955, n.p.).

Patients told the committee that the fluid-filled prostheses were heavy and they could feel the fluid moving about. Moreover, they hardened after about 18 months, which made them look unnatural (Dericks, 1954–1955). Committee members contacted multiple local New York stores to find out what types of prostheses, if any, were offered, and they experimented with the prostheses that they bought (Dericks, 1954–1955). They injected older prostheses with glycerin (which made them lumpy) and water (which helped) to make them last longer (Dericks, 1954–1955). Dericks herself visited one store where sponge rubber prosthesis were individually carved to match not only the remaining breast but to fill in the postsurgical depressions in the chest wall and the axilla (Dericks, 1954–1955). This was important because "some patients are more concerned about the 'gaps' in the axilla than the removal of the breast" (Dericks, 1954–1955, n.p.). However they also found through their interviews with patients and office nurses that the depression in the axilla lessoned after a few months. This was reassuring information they could now give their postoperative patients.

The tangible outcome of this work was a plan of care, published in 1957, for patients undergoing radical mastectomy at the New York Hospital (Dericks, 1954–1966). In addition to routine pre- and postoperative nursing care, this report shared exercises, when and how to introduce the prosthesis, engagement of the husband in the plan of his wife's care, and referral to visiting nurses for nursing care that included psychological support for the woman in her post-mastectomy world.

Reflections

In this case study, which took place almost 30 years before the Declaration of Alma-Ata, this community was practicing primary health care (PHC). In the American culture of the 1950s, gender inequities were intensified by inequities of professional caste. A diverse group of nurses, led by Virginia Dericks, set out to improve health by principles of PHC. She involved and empowered multiple partners—patients and their husbands, nurses from many fields, surgeons, primary care physicians, and department store prostheses saleswomen. Appreciating the importance of fitting into cultural norms, in this case having two matching attractive breasts, Dericks worked with the women to attain that end. Interaction was a pivotal part of the initiative as nurses talked with the patients and physicians talked with the patients' husbands. This is perhaps not how we would communicate today, but it was culturally appropriate at that time. Dericks also understood the key role of the patients' communities as she gathered information from visiting nurses and recommended that patients should be referred to them upon hospital discharge. In summary, primary health care strategies were used to address these women's social and cultural needs as they struggled with breast cancer and surgical disfigurement. One of her cancer patients (RW) later recalled, "She talked to me so nice, she gave me courage" (Dericks, 1954–1966, n.p.). Dericks gave the "right kind of care."

Community Participatory Strategies in Rural America Today

Much like the primary health care strategies described in the previous sections, public health nursing (PHN) is provided in collaboration with individuals, families, communities, and populations as well as agencies, and it is focused on population characteristics (Kulbok, Thatcher, Park, & Meszaros, 2012). Primary health care, similar to PHN, is provided with attention to the cultural context of the community or population as a whole; that is, the unique attitudinal, ecological, social, and value-based characteristics of the community or population. A model for community participation, and an exemplar of its use in a rural youth substance use prevention project, will illustrate these contemporary primary health care strategies and cultural considerations.

A Community Participatory Health Promotion Model

The community participation model (see **Figure 10-2**; Kulbok et al., 2012) is useful for PHN practice that is consistent with primary health care. The model builds on principles of community-based participatory research (CBPR), which encourages participation of community members in all processes from problem identification to project evaluation, and focuses on

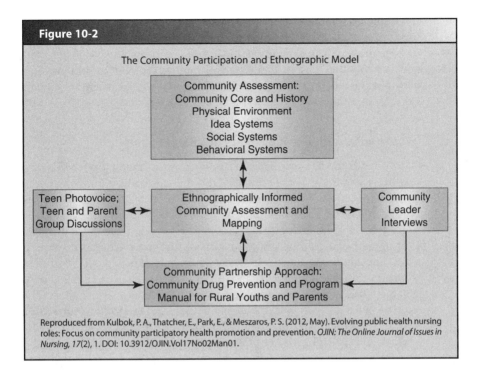

Figure 10-2

The Community Participation and Ethnographic Model

Community Assessment:
Community Core and History
Physical Environment
Idea Systems
Social Systems
Behavioral Systems

Teen Photovoice;
Teen and Parent
Group Discussions

Ethnographically Informed
Community Assessment and
Mapping

Community
Leader
Interviews

Community Partnership Approach:
Community Drug Prevention and Program
Manual for Rural Youths and Parents

Reproduced from Kulbok, P. A., Thatcher, E., Park, E., & Meszaros, P. S. (2012, May). Evolving public health nursing roles: Focus on community participatory health promotion and prevention. *OJIN: The Online Journal of Issues in Nursing, 17*(2), 1. DOI: 10.3912/OJIN.Vol17No02Man01.

community assets and resources rather than on deficits (Israel, Eng, Schulz, & Parker, 2005).

The model focuses on the cultural context of the community by utilizing local knowledge of community members and enabling public health nurses and their community partners to be sensitive to the community's cultural attitudes, beliefs, history, traditions, and values (Aronson, Wallis, O'Campo, Whitehead, & Schafer, 2007). Application of the community participation model in this exemplar includes mapping (e.g., geographic information systems [GIS]), and Photovoice (e.g., picture-taking by community members and practitioners or researchers).

GIS is useful for assessment and analysis of the cultural characteristics of a population, as well as unique aspects of phenomena of interest, such as youth substance use and nonuse in a rural community (Aronson, Wallis, O'Campo, & Schafer, 2007). Mapping enables public health nurses and their community partners to identify geographic trends over time and target interventions. With community input, maps can be generated showing where community members report protective or risk-related factors, increased or decreased substance use, and potential intervention sites. Photovoice, another useful tool to facilitate community participation, uses pictures about a given topic taken by community members to promote effective sharing of beliefs, knowledge, and thoughts through the lens of local culture (Strack, Magill, & McDonagh, 2003). For example, the rural youth culture is significant in identifying important trends in substance use or nonuse over time and for targeting interventions to high-risk rural youth. The goals of Photovoice in community participation are to enable people to record their community's assets and areas for improvement and to promote dialogue about community issues and the importance of local culture through discussion of the photographs (Kulbok et al., 2012).

Youth Substance Use Prevention in a Rural County

Rural residency has the highest rates of smoking and smokeless tobacco (ST) use, and the age of onset of smoking among youths in rural regions is earlier (American Lung Association [ALA], 2012; Shan, Jump, & Lancet, 2012). Moreover, the use of tobacco and alcohol is highly correlated (U.S. Department of Health and Humans Services [DHHS], 2007). Rural youth are at increased risk for addictions that remain untreated and may carry over into adulthood, and the potential illness burden of addiction is greater in rural areas because of lack of access to care (ALA, 2012). In the United States, tobacco use is responsible for 480,000 deaths each year, and alcohol use accounts for 88,000 deaths annually (CDC, 2014). *Healthy People 2020* (DHHS, 2010) emphasized the need to increase the number of youth who remain substance free due to the long-term health consequences of substance use. Unfortunately, many rural communities know little about intervention strategies to prevent youth substance use.

The community participation model guided an interprofessional and community team in a 3-year project to implement a substance use prevention program in a rural tobacco-growing county in the South. An advanced public health nurse and a human development specialist led the interprofessional team. The first phase of the project was to establish a community participatory research team (CPRT) made up of youth, parents, and trusted community leaders from the rural county. These individuals were committed to the project. They contributed local knowledge and an understanding of the rural youth culture in their community, which was critical to the project's success.

During the next phase, the interprofessional team and the CPRT (the team) completed a comprehensive community and environmental assessment of the rural county to identify the county's assets and needs related to five domains: people and history, physical environment, idea systems, social systems, and belief systems. In an effort to better understand the history and cultural influences of a tobacco-producing county on youth substance use or nonuse, the team completed individual interviews of community leaders, youth group interviews. and a group interview with parents. Using data from these sources and mapping strategies, the team analyzed the community assessment data related to youth substance use in the county. The team also used Photovoice to complete the community assessment the rural county. Selected youths took pictures as a visual means of collecting community and environmental assessment data that reflected both the "rural" and "youth" cultures. The photos were shown on "picture boards" according to the five domains and used to generate discussion during group interviews with youth and parents. These picture boards were then used at the end of the youth and parent group interviews to enhance each group's description of youth substance nonuse- and use-related factors in their community. (See **Figure 10-3** and **Figure 10-4** for examples from the picture board used during group interviews.)

During the next phases of the project, the team used nominal group process to evaluate and select effectiveness criteria from the research literature for youth substance use prevention programs (Winters, Fawkes, Fahnhorse, Botzet, & August, 2007). The team selected specific criteria that they felt reflected their rural county and youth culture. The team then reviewed three existing youth substance use prevention programs with effectiveness data to determine whether these programs met the selected criteria. The team matched existing programs with their selected criteria and chose Health Rocks!, a national 4-H alcohol, tobacco, and other drug use preventive program. They determined that this program was the best "fit" for their rural county based their respect for 4-H. Basic program features included

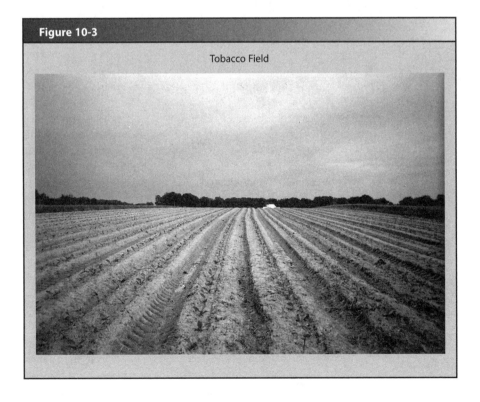

Figure 10-3

Tobacco Field

Figure 10-4

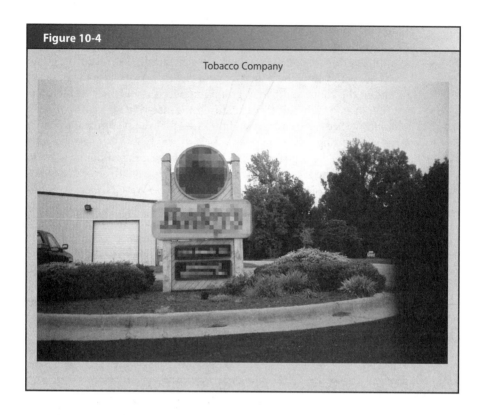

Tobacco Company

being led by a youth and adult team, easy interactive activities, and family and community level involvement (Kulbok et al., 2015).

In the final project phase, youth and adults from the rural county were trained to lead the 4-H Health Rocks! program. They implemented the program during summer school and at a summer 4-H day camp. Youth participants from the county were 10 to 17 years old; 50% were girls; 40% were in fifth grade or below; and 40% were African American. The program was successful, with more than 90% of the youth participants demonstrating positive knowledge, skills, and social competency assets related to substance use prevention at the end of the program (Kulbok et al., 2015).

Although it was challenging to maintain community participation throughout the project, the local knowledge and information learned about the unique cultural characteristics of this rural county was extremely useful for program selection and implementation. For example, the team was able to make informed decisions based on information shared between all involved including: (1) selecting middle-school-aged adolescents as the most appropriate target population for the prevention program; (2) identifying summer school and the 4-H youth camp held in the county as the most feasible and desirable settings for a youth substance use prevention program; and (3) determining that the best "instructors" for the prevention program were high school students and 4-H camp counselors, who were viewed as role models by the youth participants.

Reflections

The emphasis on collaboration and partnership between the interprofessional team and the CPRT was critical for the success of the project. In addition, this youth substance use prevention project highlights the importance of understanding the influence of cultural factors in contemporary primary health care strategies. The interplay of culture and primary health care are particularly important in the context of *Healthy People 2020* (DHHS, 2010), the ACA (2010), and Executive Order 13544 establishing the National Prevention, Health Promotion, and Public Health Council (Obama, 2010). These national initiatives provide new opportunities for culturally sensitive PHC strategies including community participation approaches that promote community health and prevention practices.

The community participation model includes long-standing PHN approaches that reflect PHC, as well as innovative strategies that public health nurses can utilize. Guided by these principles, nurses can empower communities and populations to become more involved in health promotion and prevention strategies to reduce the long-term health threats such as youth substance use. As nursing roles in primary health care evolve, greater emphasis on community participation and culturally sensitive approaches, which emphasize interprofessional collaboration, CBPR strategies, and the importance of local knowledge to address community health problems, will contribute to improved community and population health outcomes.

Conclusions

This chapter has highlighted three widely disparate underserved populations. The first two are exemplars from history and demonstrate how nurses have traditionally practiced using principles noted in PHC. The actions of these early nurses showed the use of the evolving philosophical tenets of PHC that included access of culturally sensitive and congruent care for underserved populations. The third is a contemporary model that exemplifies what we know PHC to be today. What are the themes? One could be that a community's unique culture can and should guide nurses in the provision of effective population-based PHC. Listening to these unique cultures, and actively obtaining the population's involvement, not only guides our practice but also gives necessary dignity and importance to individuals and their community—however that community is determined. Another is that although these exemplars range in time, geography, and characteristics, they all demonstrate nursing leadership and shared decision-making between nurses and communities. Use them to strengthen your professional scope.

Chapter Activities

1. Explore the determinants of health of a particular cultural group in your community that would place that group at risk.

2. Identify how you can encourage active participation of this same cultural group in the development of primary health care initiatives.

3. Identify how the full participation of this cultural group shifts the power balance in the health care system.

References

Abel, E. (1996). "We are left so much alone to work out our own problems": Nurses on American Indian Reservations during the 1930s. *Nursing History Review, 4*, 43–64.

Abel, E., & Reifel, N. (1999). Interactions between public health nurses and clients on American Indian reservations during the 1930s. In J.W. Leavitt (Ed.). *Women and Health in America* (2nd ed., pp. 489–507). Madison, WI: University of Wisconsin Press.

Affordable Care Act, read the law. (2010). Retrieved from http://www.hhs.gov /healthcare/rights/law/index.html

Alexander, S. E. (1957). Nursing care of a patient after breast surgery. *American Journal of Nursing, 57*(12), 1571–1572.

Alvord, L. A., & Van Pelt, E. C. (1999). *The scalpel and the silver bear: The first Navajo woman surgeon combines western medicine and traditional healing.* New York: Batman Books.

American Lung Association. (2012). *Cutting tobacco's rural roots: Tobacco use in rural communities.* Retrieved from http://www.lung.org/assets/documents /publications/lung-disease-data/cutting-tobaccos-rural-roots.pdf

Aronson, R. E., Wallis, A. B., O'Campo, P. J., & Schafer, P. (2007). Neighborhood mapping and evaluation: A methodology for participatory community health initiatives. *Maternal Child Health Journal, 11*, 373–383.

Aronson, R. E., Wallis, A. B., O'Campo, P. J., Whitehead, T. L., & Schafer, P. (2007). Ethnographically informed community evaluation: A framework and approach for evaluating community-based initiatives. *Maternal Child Health Journal, 11*(2), 97–109.

Bahti, M. (2000). *A Guide to Navajo sand paintings.* Tucson, AZ: Rio Nuevo Publishers.

Centers for Disease Control and Prevention. (2014). *Chronic diseases and health promotion.* Retrieved from http://www.cdc.gov/chronicdisease/overview/

Dericks, V. (1951–1958). *Mastectomy care study,* Box 2, Folder 16. Eleanor Crowder Bjoring Center for Nursing Historical Inquiry, Claude Moore Health Sciences Library, Historical Collections, University of Virginia.

Dericks, V. (1951–1967). *Mastectomy patients studied.* Box 2, Folder 15, 6.18.1951. Eleanor Crowder Bjoring Center for Nursing Historical Inquiry, Claude Moore Health Sciences Library, Historical Collections, University of Virginia.

Dericks, V. (1954–1955). *Committee.* Box 2, Folder 13, Minutes of Committee, 9.29.1954; 10.27.1954; 12.8.1954; 1.12.1955; 2.9.1955; 4.6.1955; 11.23.1955; 12.14.1955. Eleanor Crowder Bjoring Center for Nursing Historical Inquiry, Claude Moore Health Sciences Library, Historical Collections, University of Virginia.

Dericks, V. (1954–1958). *Committee to improve nursing care of mastectomy patents.* Box 2, Folder 13. Eleanor Crowder Bjoring Center for Nursing Historical Inquiry, Claude Moore Health Sciences Library, Historical Collections, University of Virginia.

Dericks, V. (1954–1966). *Notes.* Box 2, Folder 14. *Plan of care for patients undergoing radical mastectomy, The New York Hospital.* Box 2, Folder 7, October 1 1957; *RW, Colostomy care patient interviews.* Box 1, Series 2, Folder 11, 1951. Eleanor Crowder Bjoring Center for Nursing Historical Inquiry, Claude Moore Health Sciences Library, Historical Collections, University of Virginia.

Eppich, M. (1935, April). *Field nurse's narrative report*. National Archives Records Administration. RG 75, E779, box 9 [no folders], pp. 1–2.

Frisbie, C. (1987). *Navajo medicine bundles or jish: Acquisition, transmission and disposition in the past and present*. Albuquerque: University of New Mexico Press.

Forster, E. (1933, May). *Field nurse's narrative report*. National Archives Record Administration (NARA), Record Group (RG)75, E779, box 9, [no folders], pp. 1–2.

Haagensen, C. D. (1950). *Carcinoma of the breast: A monograph for the physician*. New York: American Cancer Society.

Halsted, W. S. (1894-1895). The results of operations for the cure of cancer of the breast performed at the Johns Hopkins Hospital from June 1889 to January 1894. *Johns Hopkins Hospital Report, 4*, 297–350.

Israel, B. A., Eng, E., Schulz, A. J., & Parker, E. A. (Eds.). (2005). *Methods in community-based participatory research for health*. San Francisco, CA: Jossey-Bass.

Kulbok, P. A., Meszaros, P., Bond, D., Kimbrell, M., Park, E., & Thatcher, E. (2015). Youth as partners in a community participatory project for substance use prevention. *Family & Community Health, 38*(1), 3–11.

Kulbok, P. A., Thatcher, E., Park, E., & Meszaros, P. S. (2012, May). Evolving public health nursing roles: Focus on community participatory health promotion and prevention. *OJIN: The Online Journal of Issues in Nursing, 17*(2), 1. Retrieved from http:// nursingworld.org/MainMenuCategories/ANAMarketplace/ANAPeriodicals /OJIN/TableofContents/Vol-17-2012/No2-May-2012/Evolving-Public-Health -Nursing-Roles.html

Lasser, T. (1953). *Reach for recovery*. Box 2, Folder 1, Virginia Dericks's papers. Eleanor Crowder Bjoring Center for Nursing Historical Inquiry, Claude Moore Health Sciences Library, Historical Collections, University of Virginia.

Lerner, B. H. (2001). *Breast cancer wars*. New York, NY: Oxford University Press.

Meriam, L. (1928). *The problem of Indian administration*. Baltimore, MD: The Johns Hopkins Press.

Obama, B. (2010). *Executive Order 13544—Establishing the National Prevention, Health Promotion, and Public Health Council*. Retrieved from http://www .whitehouse.gov/the-press-office/executive-order-establishing-national -prevention-health-promotion-and-public-health

Patterson, J. T. (1991). Cancer, cancerphobia, and culture. *Twentieth Century British History, 2*(2), 137–149.

Radler, H. B. (1954). *A handbook for your recovery*. Box 2, Folder 1, Virginia Dericks's papers. Eleanor Crowder Bjoring Center for Nursing Historical Inquiry, Claude Moore Health Sciences Library, Historical Collections, University of Virginia.

Renneker, R., & Cutler, M. (1952). Psychological problems of adjustment to cancer of the breast. *Journal of the American Medical Association, 148*(10), 833–838.

Seymour, N. (1935, May). *Field nurse's narrative report*. National Archives Record Administration, Record Group 75 (NARA, RG75), E779, box 9 [no folders], pp. 1–2.

Shan, M., Jump, Z., & Lancet, E. (2012). *Urban and rural disparities in tobacco use*. Retrieved from http://www.cdc.gov/nchs/ppt/nchs2012/SS-33_LANCET.pdf

Smith, G. W. (1950). When a breast must be removed. *American Journal of Nursing, 50*(6), 335–339.

Solveson, G. (1936, April). Field nurses narrative report. NARA, RG 75, box 9 (no folders), pp. 1–2.

Strack, R. W., Magill, C., & McDonagh, K. (2003). Engaging youth through photovoice. *Health Promotion Practice, 5*(1), 49–58.

Sugarbaker, E. D., & Wilfley, L. E. (1950). Cancer of the breast. *American Journal of Nursing, 50*(6), 332–335.

Trennert, R. (1998). *White man's medicine: Government doctors and the Navajo, 1863–1955.* Albuquerque: University of New Mexico Press.

U.S. Department of Health and Human Services. (2010). *Healthy people 2020.* Washington, DC: U.S. Government Printing Office.

U.S. Department of Health and Humans Services. (2007). *Alcohol alert, No. 71.* National Institutes of Health, National Institute on Alcohol Abuse and Alcoholism. Retrieved from http://pubs.niaaa.nih.gov/publications/aa71/AA71.pdf

Williams, D. (1935, August). Field nurse's narrative report. NARA, RG 75, E779, box 9 (no folders), pp. 1–2.

Winters, K. C., Fawkes, B. A., Fahnhorse, T., Botzet, A., & August, G. (2007). A synthesis review of exemplary drug abuse prevention programs in the United States. *Journal of Substance Abuse Treatment, 32,* 371–380.

Young, D. (n.d.). *Indian Health Services nursing questionnaire.* Northern Arizona University Special Collections. Virginia Brown, Ida Bahl, & Lillian Watson Collection, folder 1.4, pp. 1–2.

Zillitas, M. (n.d.). *Last Navajo assignment.* Original manuscript, MS 269, Virginia Brown, Ida Bahl, & Lillian Watson Collection, box 1, folder 1.4.

Chapter 11

Community-Based Participatory Research and Primary Health Care: Working with the People

Carol Roye and Marie Truglio-Londrigan

This chapter presents the use of a specific research method—community-based participatory research (CBPR)—that synergistically supports and enacts the concepts of primary health care. It does so by engaging those in the community as partners in the research process, allowing their perspectives to be heard and to direct the research. This method embraces the population and brings their ideas to the forefront. Seen more as a "bottom-up" approach to research, CBPR creates a climate for collaboration (Wallace, 1987). CBPR creates a shift in the power balance toward empowerment of participating community members who are seen as valued and respected partners in the research process (Baum, MacDougall, & Smith, 2006, p. 854). In addition, the attainment of knowledge and skills enhances the social capital of community participants. The chapter begins with a case study reflecting coauthor Carol Roye's experience as a pediatric nurse practitioner (PNP) and recognition of the value CBPR could bring to her practice and research in reproductive health care to the adolescent community. The process of CBPR is described in the context of how this research exemplifies the ideas of primary health care (PHC).

The Interaction Between Research and Practice: A Personal Perspective

I started practicing as a pediatric nurse practitioner (PNP) in the late 1980s in the Bronx, New York, and Upper Manhattan—two impoverished communities. The HIV/AIDS epidemic had recently been identified. As I started my clinical practice, I was not concerned about HIV for my patients because at first it was believed to be a disease exclusively of men who have sex with men. Over time, however, it became clear that women were contracting the disease, especially poor women of color like those I was caring for. I became concerned that my patients, who were all sexually active teens and many of whom were already mothers, were at risk for HIV. Moreover, I gave each of them a prescription for hormonal contraception, usually birth control pills. I wondered whether having the pills made them less likely to use condoms. If I did not give them the prescription, I worried that they would have sex without condoms or pills and be at higher risk for pregnancy and HIV. To better understand this population, I did a quantitative study with more than 600 adolescent and young adult women from the community. I found that, indeed, young women who use hormonal contraception are less likely to use condoms than those who do not (Roye, 1998). Knowing this, it was important to intervene in a way that would be meaningful to the young women and would encourage their use of condoms.

I realized, over time, that I had to turn to the young women for the answers. I studied these behaviors in my doctoral program, and I could speculate about the answer. But I am not a young woman from their community, and nothing I learned from books could adequately answer the question. Therefore, I turned to the "experts," the young women themselves, listening to and hearing their voices. In a qualitative study, we asked them about their condom use and nonuse. For example, they were asked to complete this sentence: "The last time I had sex and used a condom, I used a condom because...." The young women told us things we never would have thought to ask about, such as that they did not use a condom because they "trusted" their partner or because they "had been together all week." In addition, we asked the young women what we could do to help teenage girls like them reduce their HIV risk behaviors. They told us that it would be helpful to see young women who look like them who have HIV. If they saw that, they felt it would make an impression on them and prompt them to use condoms. These insights contextualized their experiences and their perceptions about what teens needed to both know and see to understand that indeed they were at risk for HIV.

These insights were the basis for development of an HIV-prevention program, which featured a video showing HIV-infected women. We also included an interactive counseling program that had been effective with adults. Thus, we developed and tested a program to promote dual method use (condom and hormonal method) by sexually active young women. I received funding, developed a video called *Reality Check*, adapted an HIV-prevention counseling protocol called Project RESPECT (Kamb et al., 1998), and tested the efficacy of the video in a randomized clinical trial (Roye, Perlmutter Silverman, & Krauss, 2007). The video was based on many of the insights the teens had provided during the interviews, which is why it features HIV-positive young women. For the new study, teens were randomized to one of four groups: (1) watch the video only, (2) counseling only, (3) video followed by counseling, and (4) usual care with no special intervention. We gave an extensive behavioral questionnaire before the young women participated in the intervention, and again 3 months after the intervention. We found that the young women who had seen the video and then received counseling were significantly more likely to report condom use than young women in the other groups, demonstrating that the video and counseling were effective at promoting condom use.

Since this time I have integrated the knowledge learned from my research into my practice and educational endeavors. We subsequently added the counseling protocol to the video, and it is now being used across the nation in HIV-prevention programs. If any researcher developed a prevention program for teens to reduce their risk of any behaviorally associated health problem, such as drug use or smoking, without their input, it is likely that the program would be less effective than it would be with their input. Furthermore, since this time I have come to see that the involvement of the people at all levels of the research process, such as in CBPR, would be beneficial on many levels. For example, if I had met with the adolescent girls in my practice sooner in the research planning process, the interventions could have been more meaningful for them from the beginning, rather than being based on what I assumed the results might be. Primary health care in our nation is a work in progress, and I have learned that one way I can act to move the nation forward toward PHC is by including the people affected as partners in the research process from inception to evaluation.

I had not read about CBPR when I began doing studies with the young women who were the target vulnerable population for my studies, so this is not an example of CBPR. I began to be introduced to CBPR as I realized that if I had these vulnerable teens and the community partner with me in the initial research endeavor from its inception, the research would develop and unfold very differently along the way. Perhaps most important, the personal experience of these young teens as they participated would be vastly different.

Community-Based Participatory Research

CBPR focuses on inequities through the active involvement of the people in the community (Israel, Schulz, Parker, & Becker, 1998). According to Hills, Mullett, and Carroll (2007):

> CBPR is a planned, systematic approach to issues relevant to the target community, requires community involvement in the research, has a

problem-solving focus, is directed at societal change, and makes a lasting contribution to the community.... The issues are identified by the people who have an interest or stake in it, and these stakeholders participate in all aspects of the research process. (p. 127)

Katz (2015) further expands upon this and sees CBPR not as a method but as an approach to research whereby the principles of CBPR embody "a democratic, community-centered, capacity building and action-oriented process for positive change—mak[ing] it a good fit for communities" (p. 151). A visual presentation of CBPR (see **Figure 11-1***)* appears simple in design, yet the actual process is complex, with multiple layers requiring reflective practice throughout. The process begins with the community partnership initiation, development, and the recognition of strategies to sustain the partnership. Once the partnership is developed, the additional phases unfold. These phases include planning, action, reflection, and evaluation/ review (Breda, 2015; Kelly, 2005). Dissemination is also an important phase to consider in the CBPR. A more detailed explanation of each of these phases follows.

A Partnership Built on Trust

The foundation of CBPR is acknowledging that emphasis must be placed squarely in the community and within the community. It is the researcher who must gain access to the community; after all it is called community-based for a very important reason. Gaining access into the community is a complex task that will vary from community to community and depend on the history of that community. If the researcher has some established connections to the community—for example, if a school of nursing has students involved in clinical experiences there—a relationship and trust may already be in evidence. In other situations, the researcher may know key individuals or organizations within the community. As a result of these trust-based relationships, the researcher may be able to reach into that community with greater ease to introduce the notion of developing formal connections to carry out a CBPR. It is important to remember that trust is essential at the beginning of the CBPR process (Whyte, 1989). This may not always be the case, and researchers will need to carefully "think" of ways to gain entry into the community and develop participatory relationships (White, Suchowier-ska, & Campbell, 2004). Building trust and respect is necessary so that collaboration and equality of participatory action is embraced, fostered, and sustained over time.

These beginning steps were in evidence in the CBPR carried out by Gallagher, Truglio-Londrigan, and Levin (2009), who wanted to partner with a town just northeast of New York City and develop a project for older adults residing in the community. The researchers had gathered initial data and noted that the town's population was aging. They wanted to partner for

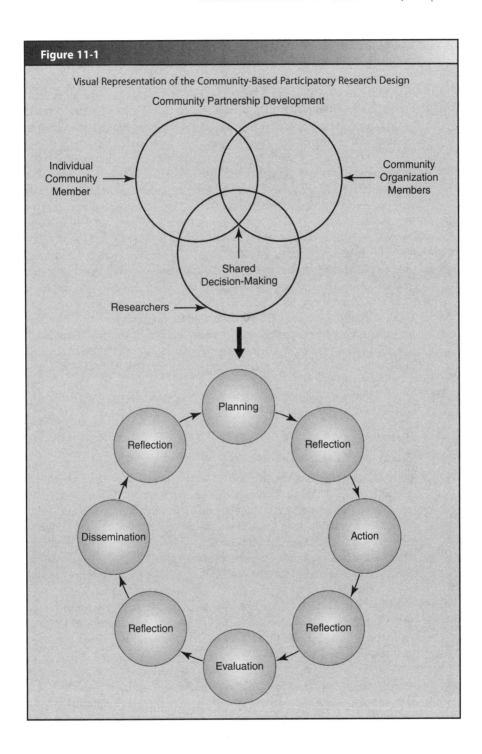

Figure 11-1

Visual Representation of the Community-Based Participatory Research Design

two purposes: (1) to establish a *Partnership for Healthy Living* so individuals could age successfully in place, and (2) to carry out this project via the CBPR. The success of this program and the potential for positive health outcomes rested with gaining the knowledge and guidance of the older adult partners who would share their lived experiences, thereby strengthening the program design, implementation, and dissemination. The researchers first contacted the town mayor, who happened to be a nurse and a very strong ally. The town mayor was a trusted member of the community; she was a longtime resident and her father had also been town mayor in the past. The mayor introduced the researchers to the Town Nutrition Center, which was the place chosen for the *Partnership for Healthy Living* because the mayor noted it was a gathering place for the community dwelling older adults. The mayor introduced the researchers to the older adults who came to the nutrition site and to the professionals at the site. Before the researchers approached the older adults about the CBPR, the professionals suggested that the researchers "spend time" at the site so the older adults would come to "know" and "connect" with them. This did in fact take place. The researchers worked with the older adults, and together they developed a series of educational programs suggested by the older adults. These first steps were essential in establishing a strong foundational beginning that strengthened the partnership between the community members and the researchers. It also enhanced the researchers' "ability to identify, understand, and effectively address the issues" (Hill, Mullett, & Carroll, 2007, p. 126).

Planning

Planning is described as taking place as a separate and distinct step in the research process; however, it really is an important step throughout the research process. For example, planning determines what data need to be gathered for an assessment and how to collect that information, and this involves all individuals in the CBPR. Identifying problems and setting priorities is also a collaborative, shared decision by all members of the CBPR. Once researchers identify the problem and make a shared decision about the intervention to address the problem, further planning provides strategies to best deliver the interventions and by whom. Planning determines what additional information needs to be gathered and by whom for the evaluation process and dissemination of the research results. Foster, Chiang, Hillard, Hall, and Heath (2010) show us an example of the planning process as it relates to the assessments.

Once the relationship is established between the researchers and the community of individuals and organizations, a community assessment is conducted to identify the strengths and weaknesses of that community. The researchers may be experts in the formal, systematic ways of gathering information, but the community participants know their community and will add important information related to the best ways to access and gather the needed data. For example, who are the key informants in the community, how can they be reached, and who will make the introductions so that these key informants feel they can trust the interviewer and ultimately be at ease? In some CBPR, a person from the community may be engaged to help in the community assessment and may conduct the interviews. Foster and colleagues (2010) were members of a cross-cultural team, which consisted of U.S. midwife researchers, Dominican nurses, and community leaders. A CBPR project was embarked on because Dominican nurses had witnessed pregnant women not accessing care when needed, resulting in poor health outcomes and death. The CBPR research team included a community health worker (CHW). These CHWs proved invaluable in gathering information throughout the research process. One such example was the formation of small groups, called little brigades, which were comprised of the CHW, a nurse, and a U.S. researcher/assistant. These brigades went out into the neighborhoods, knocking on doors to recruit women for focus groups. The CHWs also made observations about the prenatal care process and how prenatal care was a deterrent to health. The CHWs engaged in note taking about the prenatal care process, identifying problems and the inherent lack of quality and comfort. Their insider perspective in gathering data was invaluable to the research process.

It is important to recognize that researchers may already have an idea about the needs of a particular community and population, and this idea may have been the original reason to take the early steps to enter a community. A comprehensive community assessment that involves gathering additional data in a systematic way, including using large data sets and analyzing that data for population-based trends, is still important (Kelly, 2005). The end result of this assessment may mean that the information gathered is not what the researchers initially thought. Or, it is also possible that the community of individuals will raise questions that lead to alternative yet important conversations about the data being gathered. The outside researchers must remember that the individuals, who have the experience of living within the specified community, may offer additional insights that the data from the large data sets do not reveal. The important point is that every person is given the opportunity to speak and to be heard. The action of speaking and being heard models, for the individuals within the community, that no one person has power over any individual and that the power is deliberately shared between the researchers and the individuals in the community who are participating in the CBPR (Baum et al., 2006). Ultimately, the outcome of the community and population-based collaborative assessment is to identify the vulnerable population and the primary issue of this population. In addition, the determinants of health that place this population at further risk are collaboratively and collectively decided. The remainder of the research process is based on this final determination.

Action

The action phase begins with questions that are important for planning the action. As in the planning phase, the researchers may have expertise in carrying out a formal, systematic review to identify best practice for the issue identified from the assessment. Again, there are conversations about the interventions, because the community people know and understand the ideas, values, and beliefs of the people and will offer valuable insight. Remembering the importance of patient and population preferences, the researchers listen and hear. The types of interventions initiated and the strategies that will be used to initiate these interventions are explored in questions like these:

- What is the intervention that the people see as important?
- What strategy will be used to deliver the intervention?
- Who is the best person to deliver the intervention?
- When is the best time to deliver the intervention?
- Where is the best location for implementation?

These types of questions and the answers signal the importance of community member participation. Who but an individual living in the targeted community would know the specific answers to these questions so that interventions are culturally congruent?

Let's look at an HIV-prevention program for heterosexual Black men in Brooklyn that took place in barbershops (Wilson et al., 2014). The study community was an area with a high prevalence of HIV and AIDS. The goal of the project was to improve the men's skills and motivation to decrease their own risk from their sexual behaviors, as well as to build their desire and capacity to improve the health of their community (Wilson et al., 2014). The researchers began by creating a steering committee composed of health professionals, barbers, a pastor, and men from the community (an area with a high HIV-prevalence). Even though the professionals in this group all had worked in the community for years and knew community members well, they realized they needed the actual voices of community members at the table to design the most effective prevention intervention. The steering committee suggested approaches to addressing all aspects of the program, from giving it a name, to the details of recruitment, retention, evaluation, and the intervention itself. The team collected quantitative and qualitative data to inform the content of the intervention. Focus groups and interviews with community men, aged 18 to 45, covered relevant topics including masculinity, partner selection, sexual risk behaviors, myths and stigma around HIV, and suggestions for program development. Trust and higher emotional attachment emerged as themes during data analysis, as well as a low perceived risk of HIV and concerns about discussing safer sex with long-term partners. The men also spoke of the need for HIV-prevention programming to originate from trusted sources in the community (Wilson et al., 2014).

Evaluation

In the evaluation phase, participants evaluate what was done and how it was done, and determine whether or not their goals and outcomes were achieved. The evaluation phase of the CBPR process also provides an opportunity for an evaluation of "other" outcomes that may have been witnessed and experienced by the community members who were collaborators in the research process. For example, Ochocka, Janenz, and Nelson (2002) identified that both formal and informal learning opportunities take place during the research process for both the researchers and the members from the community. Additional outcomes of CBPR include empowerment of all individuals and the community. Van der Velde, Williamson, and Ogilvie (2010) describe CBPR community participant researchers as gaining:

> confidence by having their internal knowledge validated (the knowledge they brought to the initiative), by learning and practicing new skills (the knowledge they gained because of their involvement) and by witnessing changes in other participants and themselves. These experiences fueled further involvement and led to a sense of personal empowerment. (p. 1300)

Dissemination

Dissemination is important to the entire research process. Frequently, researchers see dissemination as the publication and presentation of research outcomes. CBPR expands this understanding to take on additional meaning. How can we as researchers ensure that changes do come about as an outgrowth of our research efforts and become embedded in the fabric of the community we are serving? One way to answer this question is to look at ways and means to make system changes. The Minnesota Department of Health Division of Community Health Services Public Health Nursing Section (2001) published *Public Health Interventions: Applications for Public Health Nursing Practice,* which provides an extensive description and explanation of the interventions public health nurses take on in their work with individuals, families, communities, and populations. This information is visually presented in the form of a model that demonstrates interventions applied by public health nurses at three identified levels of practice: community-focused practice, system-focused practice, and individual-focused practice (pp. 4–5). Public health nursing interventions that take place at the system-focused practice are interventions focused on organizations, policies, and laws thereby facilitating a dissemination that reaches a broader audience with greater effectiveness and "a long-lasting way to impact population health...." (p. 5). Dissemination is an important aspect of the research process for it both assures the population and ensures that the work of the CBPR process will be felt in the community as system changes in the form of policies and laws. For example, the work of the Allies Against Asthma

Coalition illustrates how dissemination of research findings through policy and system change can lead to better health outcomes. This coalition, supported by the Robert Wood Johnson Foundation, was successful in the facilitation of policy and system change at institutional levels and in statewide legislation changes that resulted in better health outcomes (Clark et al., 2010).

Reflection

Reflection is a process of discovery and is an important part of CBPR. This discovery signals an inquiry in and of itself where those who participate are enhancing their understanding of the experience they are living so that their practice, in this case the research process, may be improved upon (Baum et al., 2006). Koch, Mann, Kralik, and van Loon (2005) describe the reflective process as involving the "look, think and act cycles" central to participatory research. Schön (2006) identified the process of reflection-in-action and reflection-on-action. Reflection-in-action takes place as health care providers, in this case the researchers, "think about what we are doing" (p. 54) while doing it. And while the researchers and the community of participants are individually and collectively thinking about what they are doing, they are "evolving their way of doing it" (p. 56). Reflection-on-action takes place after the interaction, as the health care provider and/or community of researchers "thinks back on a project they have undertaken, a situation they have lived through, and they explore the understandings they have brought to their handling of the case" (p. 61). For example, the process of individual researchers or a community of researchers taking field notes in CBPR can serve as a point of reflection-on-action at a later moment in time, which enhances the research process. This is seen in the work of Ochocka, Janzen, and Nelson (2002), who engaged in research with consumer/survivors with mental health problems, and also in the work of Conder, Milner, and Mirfin-Veitch (2011), who worked with individuals with intellectual disabilities. An important part of their research was note taking, which fostered moments of reflection.

The reflective process takes place on multiple levels, including individual self-reflective questioning, collective reflective questioning involving the entire CBPR community members, and the collective reflective questioning that pertains to the research process. Questions that represent each of these levels are listed in **Table 11-1**. These are just a few of the reflective questions participants involved in the CBPR process may engage.

Ethical Considerations

Ethical considerations are recognized in CBPR as in any other research approach, but specific challenges inherent in CBPR need to be considered. Jones and Gelling (2013) identify one of the main challenges of this type of

Table 11-1

Reflective Process and Questions

Reflective Process	Reflective Questions
Individual Self-Reflective Questioning	• Am I prepared to work with the people from the community? • How do I feel about working in a collaborative partnership? • Am I comfortable with shifting the balance of power? • How do I relate and respond to others? • How do others relate and respond to me?
Community Members Collective Reflective Questioning	• Does the group feel as though they can express their ideas, values, and beliefs with ease? • Does the group feel that each person is given the opportunity to speak? • Does the group feel that each person is listened to and heard? • Does each member of the group feel valued and respected? • Does each member of the group feel satisfied with the process?
Community Members Collective Reflective Questioning About the CBPR Process	• Has the assessment process been carried out in a systematic and comprehensive way and acknowledged and integrated community members suggestions? • Do all members believe that the data collected is accurate, and has the voice of the people in the community been heard? • Have community members been involved in data collection? • How did the people who live in the community respond to those carrying out the assessment? • Were all members in agreement with the outcomes of the assessment in terms of the population and population-based issue identified? • How was the intervention identified? Was it based in best practice? If the community identified that the evidence was not in line with the population's preference and beliefs, how was this addressed? What were the outcomes of these discussions? • How was the intervention delivered and by whom? Was there consideration for cultural congruence? • How was the evaluation process instituted, and were the community members involved? • Has the dissemination process been successful? • Were adequate resources available throughout the process, such as educational programming to support those involved in learning how to work collaboratively, communication, conflict resolution and negotiation, finances, technology, availability of consultations, and managerial support?

Data from Foster, J., Chiang, F., Hillard, R. C., Hall, P., & Heath, A. (2010). Team process in community-based participatory research on maternity care in the Dominican Republic. *Nursing Inquiry, 17*(4), 309–316.

Kelly, P. (2005). Practical suggestions for community interventions using participatory action research. *Public Health Nursing,* 22(1), 65–73.

Truglio-Londrigan, M. (2015). Participatory action research: one researcher's reflection. In M. de Chesnay (Ed.), Nursing research using participatory action research (pp, 117-135), New York: Springer Publishing Company.

White, G. W., Suchowieska, M., & Campbell, M. (2004). Developing and systematically implementing participatory action research. *Archives of Physical Medicine and Rehabilitation,* 85(Suppl. 2), s3–s12.

research as attainment of institutional review board approval. Researchers need to concisely and comprehensively document the project and how it will be carried out before community partnerships have been fully established. Additional challenges have been noted by Bromley, Mikesell, Jones, and Khodyakov (2015), who carried out interviews with community and academic researchers to obtain their perspectives on ethical challenges in community-engaged research. Based on these interviews, four key principles were identified that described ethical community-engaged research: embody ethical action, respect participants, generalize beneficence, and negotiate justice (p. 903). Challenges were associated with each of these key principles. For example, the interviewees saw embodying ethical action as "actualizing a new type of ethical practice through mutuality, equity, and shared responsibility. These were valued ends in themselves—not just means to knowledge production" (p. 902). In addition, the interviewees viewed the principle of respect for participants in a much broader way. These interviewees sought to "practice respect, truthfulness, and free choice with enrolled and potential participants, research partners, study site staff, community members, and the community as a whole" (Bromley et al., 2015, p. 903). These four principles demonstrate the expansive nature of ethical challenges faced by the researchers, with both academic and community members highlighting the importance of reflection and communication throughout the research process.

Conclusion and Reflections on Primary Health Care

The Declaration of Alma-Ata (WHO, 1978) addresses the need for communities to participate as major stakeholders in planning, organizing, and operating initiatives toward self-reliance and the attainment of health. *People at the Centre of Health Care: Harmonizing Mind and Body, People and Systems* (WHO, 2007) begins to address the idea of putting people at the center of health care. This idea is further explicated in *Primary Health Care: Now More Than Ever* (WHO, 2008). CBPR exemplifies this value by placing people at the center and is a model of PHC in action. It is a way of conducting research with collaboration between all involved, including the people in the community, and understanding the importance each individual and community organization brings to the CBPR process. Nolan and Grant (1993) see this approach as different from the traditional "top-down" way of conducting research. Rather, the value of action research is in its bottom-up approach, which creates a climate for collaboration (Wallace, 1987). By extension, involvement in CBPR creates a shift in the power balance toward empowerment, which is experienced by participating community members as their lived experiences now include being valued, respected, listened to, and heard as the "researched cease to be objects and become partners in the whole research process" (Baum et al., 2006, p. 854). In addition, knowledge and skills learned enhance the community participants own capital. Ultimately, CBPR is a process that facilitates personal change and has the potential to lead to societal change. After all, "[s]ocial change cannot occur without personal change" (van der Velde, Williamson, & Ogilvie, 2010, p. 1299).

Chapter Activities

1. Delve into the library databases and search for community-based participatory research (CBPR) studies. Once you have found an article, identify what made the research process community-based and participatory in nature. Based on your careful review, can you suggest additional ways the people in the community could be further engaged throughout the research process?

2. Can you identify some individual self-reflective questions or community member collective reflective questions beyond those listed in Table 11-1?

3. How does CBPR mirror the essential elements of primary health care?

4. Explore how Carol Roye's work with this vulnerable adolescent population could have been developed into a study using CBPR to better connect with the issues of this population. In what ways could the outcomes have been different?

References

Baum, F., MacDougall, C., & Smith, D. (2006). Participatory action research. *Journal of Epidemiology and Community Health, 60*(10), 854–857.

Breda, K. L. (2015). Participatory action research. In M. De Chesnay (Ed.), *Nursing research using participatory action research* (pp. 1-11), New York, NY: Springer Publishing Company.

Bromley, E., Mikesell, L., Jones, F., & Khodyakov, D. (2015). From subject to participant: Ethics and the evolving role of community health research. *American Journal of Public Health, 105*(5), 900–908.

Clark, J. (2003). Furore erupts over NIH "hit list." *British Medical Journal, 327*, 1065.

Clark, N. C., Lachance, L., Doctor, L. J., Gilmore, L., Kelly, C., et al. (2010). Policy and System Change and Community Coalitions: Outcomes From Allies Against Asthma. *American Journal of Public Health, 100* (5), 904-912. (doi: 10.2105/AJPH.2009.180869). Retrieved from http://ajph.aphapublications.org/doi/full/10.2105/AJPH.2009.180869

Conder, J., Milner, P., & Mirfin-Veitch, B. (2011). Reflections on a participatory project: The rewards and challenges for the lead researchers. *Journal of Intellectual & Developmental Disability, 36*(1), 39–48.

Foster, J., Chiang, F., Hillard, R. C., Hall, P., & Heath, A. (2010). Team process in community-based participatory research on maternity care in the Dominican Republic. *Nursing Inquiry, 17*(4), 309–316.

Gallagher, L., Truglio-Londrigan, M., & Levin, R. (2009). Partnership for healthy living: An action research project. *Nurse Researcher, 16*(2), 7–29.

Hills, M., Mullett, J., & Carroll, S. (2007). Community-based participatory action research: Transforming multidisciplinary practice in primary health care. *American Journal of Public Health, 21*(2/3), 125–135.

Israel, B. A., Schulz, A. J., Parker, E. A., & Becker, A. B. (1998). Review of community-based research: Assessing partnership approaches to improve public health. *Annual Review of Public Health, 19*, 173–202.

Jones, S., & Gelling, L. (2013). Participation in action research. *Nurse Researcher, 21*(2), 6–7.

Kamb, M. L., Fishbein, M., Douglas, J. M., Jr., Rhodes, F., Rogers, J., Bolan, G., et al. (1998). Efficacy of risk-reduction counseling to prevent human immunodeficiency virus and sexually transmitted diseases: A randomized controlled trial. Project RESPECT study group. *Journal of the American Medical Association, 280*(13), 1161–1167.

Katz, J. (2015). A university-tribal community-based participatory research partnership: Determining community priorities for the health of youth. In M. De Chesnay (Ed.), *Nursing research using participatory action research* (pp. 151–160), New York, NY: Springer Publishing Company.

Kelly, P. (2005). Practical suggestions for community interventions using participatory action research. *Public Health Nursing, 22*(1), 65–73.

Koch, T., Mann, S., Kralik, D., & van Loon, A. M. (2005). Reflection: look, think and act cycles in participatory action research. *Journal of Nursing Research, 10*(3), 261–277.

Minnesota Department of Health Division of Community Health Services Public Health Nursing Section. (2001). *Public health interventions: applications for public health nursing practice*. Author: Minnesota.

Nolan, M., & Grant, G. (1993). Action research and quality of care: A mechanism for agreeing basic values as a precursor to change. *Journal of Advanced Nursing, 18*(2), 305–311.

Ochocka, J., Janzen, R., & Nelson, G. (2002). Sharing power and knowledge: Professional and mental health consumer/survivor researchers working together in a participatory action research project. *Psychiatric Rehabilitation Journal, 25*(4), 379–387.

Public Health Nursing Section: Public Health Interventions. (2001). *Applications for public health nursing practice*. St. Paul: Minnesota Department of Health.

Roye, C. F. (1998). Condom use by Hispanic and African-American adolescent girls who use hormonal contraception. *Journal of Adolescent Health, 23*(4), 205–211.

Roye, C., Perlmutter Silverman, P., & Krauss, B. (2007). A brief, low-cost, theory-based intervention to promote dual method use by Black and Latina female adolescents: A randomized clinical trial. *Health Education & Behavior: The Official Publication of the Society for Public Health Education, 34*(4), 608–621.

Schön, D. (2006). *The reflective practitioner: How professionals think in action*. Aldershot, England: Ashgate Publishing Limited.

Truglio-Londrigan, Marie. (2015). Participatory action research: one researcher's reflection. In M. De Chesnay (Ed.), *Nursing research using participatory action research* (pp, 117-135), New York, NY: Springer Publishing Company.

Van der Velde, J., Williamson, D. L., & Ogilvie, L. D. (2010). Participatory action research: Practical strategies for actively engaging and maintaining participation in immigrant refugee communities. *Qualitative Health Research, 19*(9), 1293–1302.

Wald, L. (1918). *Public health nursing*. Unpublished speech to be read at the Pan-American Congress on Child Welfare. New York, NY: New York Public Library, Lillian Wald papers, reel 25, pp. 1–12.

Wallace, M. (1987). A historical review of action research: some implications for the education of teachers in their managerial role. *Journal of Education for Teaching, 13*(2), 97–110.

White, G. W., Suchowieska, M., & Campbell, M. (2004). Developing and systematically implementing participatory action research. *Archives of Physical Medicine and Rehabilitation, 85*(Suppl. 2), s3–s12.

Whyte, W. F. (1989). Advancing scientific knowledge through participatory action research. *Sociological Forum, 4*(3), 367–385.

Wilson, T. E., Fraser-White, M., Williams, K. M., Pinto, A., Agbetor, F., Camilien, B., et al. (2014). Barbershop talk with brothers: Using community-based participatory research to develop and pilot test a program to reduce HIV risk among Black heterosexual men. *AIDS Education and Prevention: Official Publication of the International Society for AIDS Education, 26*(5), 383–397.

World Health Organization. (1978). *Declaration of Alma-Ata*. Retrieved from http://www.who.int/publications/almaata_declaration_en.pdf?ua=1

World Health Organization. (2007). *Placing people at the centre of health care: Harmonizing mind and body, people and systems*. Geneva, Switzerland: Author.

World Health Organization. (2008). *Primary health care: Now more than ever*. Geneva, Switzerland: Author.

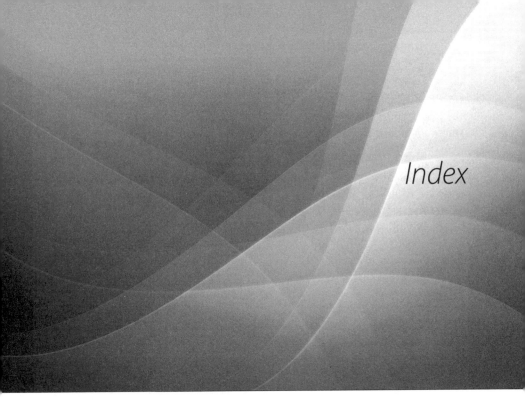

Index

Federal Trade Commission, 115–116
Federally Qualified Health Center, 126
Feighery, E., 91
FHBC. *See* Family Health and
  Birth Center
FNPs. *See* family nurse practitioners
FNS. *See* Frontier Nursing Service
Foley, Edna, 90
Forster, Elizabeth, 163, 165
Foster, J., 186–187
Foster-Fishman, P. G., 102
freestanding birth center, 119–122
Frey, D., 100
Frontier Nursing Service (FNS), 111
The Future of Nursing: Leading Change,
  Advancing Health (IOM), 45

G

Gallagher, L., 184
GBD. *See* global burden of disease
Gehlert, S., 70
geographic information systems
  (GIS), 171
GIS. *See* geographic information systems
Global Alliance for Leadership in
  Nursing Education and Science, 147
global burden of disease (GBD)
  leading causes of, 146f
  MDGs and, 143–144
global health
  case studies on, 151–155
  collaboration needed for, 142, 155
  meetings to advance, 150
  nurses contribution to, 151, 155
  PHC in, 151–155
  strategy for, 143
global health competencies, 147,
  148t–149t
global nurse
  education and competencies of,
  146–150
  skills and knowledge of, 149–150
  Supercourse website for, 147

Gluckman, Henry, 22
Goff, D. C., 127
Government and Community Alliances,
  Hartford Hospital and, 93–94
grassroots coalition, 91
Greitemeyer, T., 100

H

Haiti, PHC mission, 152–153
Hall, P., 186–187
A Handbook for Your Recovery
  (Radler), 167
Harrison, Esther, 14, 15
Hartford Healthcare System, 93
Hartford Hospital
  Black Men's Health Project and, 94
  Government and Community
    Alliances and, 93–94
  health disparities experienced by,
    93–94
  partnerships developed by, 94
Hartsfeld, Veronica, 121–122
HBP. *See* Healthy Babies Project
health behavior, nursing interventions
  for, 68
health care finance, 79–80
health care policy, 2, 63
health care spending, 79
  ACA impacting, 80
  lowering of, 82
  nursing and, 80–81
  per capita cost reduction in, 76
  in United States, 80
health disparities, 65, 93–94
health equality, 65
health inequalities
  advocacy and, 67
  health disparities compared to, 65
  reduction of, 65, 69–70
Health Provider Shortage Areas
  (HPSAs), 133
Health Resources and Services
  Administration (HRSA), 133